Eating to Win

with America's #1 Food Coach

Eating to Win

with America's #1 Food Coach

Majid "Magic" Noori
with Skip Anderson and Fred DuBose

ETW Partnership

Nashville • New York

Acknowledgements

It is with grateful appreciation that Magic Noori thanks those who have encouraged him during the process of writing this book, most notably his wife and daughter, his coauthors, his very capable and eternally patient editorial assistant Katie Harp Pratt, the thousands of student athletes with whom he has worked, the dozens of those whose talents carried them to the professional ranks, and the coaches and administrators at Vanderbilt University. And, of course, the incomparable Tammy Boclair. Skip Anderson is the founding editor of *Commodore Nation*, the official magazine for Vanderbilt University's athletics. He thanks his sister, April, for her love, Craig and Richard Fontaine for their encouragement, Mark Reagan and Jules Childress for their patience, and Mike Schoenfeld and Beth Fortune for their support. Fred DuBose thanks his decades-long career as a developer and editor of Reader's Digest practical books of all stripes.

ISBN 978-1470059927

Table of Contents

My Road to the Training Table

That you're reading *Eating to Win* probably means you play sports of some sort, run marathons, or simply believe energetic physical activity is the road to health and happiness. You could be an 18-year-old who plays on your high school football or basketball team or a middle-aged "weekend warrior" who hits the tennis court or golf course now and then. You could be a grandparent determined to get in an hour of walking each day to keep your heart strong and your weight steady. Or you might even be among those select few who've entered the hallowed realm of professional sports. Whatever the case, you live a physically active life, and you like it.

With all of the media attention given to fitness, you no doubt know that a long-term food plan – as opposed to a few weeks' effort to lose weight and stay fit – is part of a winning strategy. And because you love getting physical, what better food plan to adopt (and adapt) than one tailored to athletes?

That's what I do for a living, and the Training Table model I've developed over the years can be your ticket not only to improving your performance on the field or track but also to maintaining your optimum weight and fitness level.

From Swimming to Sports Nutrition

In my youth I was a competitive swimmer in Iran, and after a while I realized there was a connection between what I ate and how I well I swam. It wasn't just what I'd eaten the night before that affected my performance but also the food I'd had in the days leading up to competitions. What's more, it dawned on me how vital being well rested was to peak performance in the pool, and that *when* I rested also mattered.

This realization inspired a passion to help other athletes and propelled me to a degree in nutrition and sports science from the University of Tehran. My move to the United States in 1977 led to a successful career as a chef in Nashville, Tennessee, and in 1990 Vanderbilt University recruited me to cook for the men and women of their then fourteen (now sixteen) athletic teams. I jumped at the chance and quickly devised a "training table" program. Here's a glimpse of the game plan in its infancy:

In the summer of 1991 I loaded up my fledgling Training Table and moved it to the nearby hamlet of Bell Buckle, then the site of the Vanderbilt Commodores football training camp. Many players worried they would lose needed poundage – not surprising, given the two-a-days in the South's scorching heat. So the coaches and I worked together to beat the odds: They made sure the players' practice schedules allowed ample time for resting and eating, and I kept the right food coming.

By the end of the training, almost all of the players had either maintained their weight or added muscle. Before long they recognized the power of thinking beyond hunger and habit – and I caught the attention of *Sports Illustrated*, which called my nutrition program the best in college football. The magazine later chronicled its progress time after time and named me "Food Coach of the Year."

Today my Training Table serves more than 300 Vanderbilt Commodores and is the model for other colleges striving to give their athletes a competitive edge. In addition, I've helped young men and women outside the university take their game to the next level – among them, high school athletes and more than a few Tennessee Titans.

Go For It!

At its core, the Training Table program is rooted in my winning formula of FREE – Food/Fluids, Rest, Exercise, and Education, as explained in Chapter 1. What has worked for the athletes I've advised – whether they play for the NFL, NBA, NHL, Major League Baseball or as enthusiastic amateurs – can also work for *you*. Developing a personal program requires discipline and resolve, of course. But once you get into the habit of approaching food and drink by way of the Training Table, you're home free. Enjoy reading *Eating to Win*, and good luck!

– Majid "Magic" Noori

January 2012

––– *Take Note* –––

Playing Hardball with Soft Drinks

I work very closely with Vanderbilt athletes, both in the Hendrix Dining Room and during summer training.

And from the beginning, they've known that I'm bull-headed when it comes to changing eating habits. In fact, on the first day of my job in 1990, I pulled the plug on the dining room's soft drink machine. The typical cola gives you nothing more than empty calories, way too much sugar, and – perhaps worst of all – a big dose of dehydrating caffeine. In short, soft drinks are counterproductive to an your progress toward peak performance.

After disabling the machine, I called the vending company and asked that it be removed. After days passed and it became obvious the company was ignoring me, I informed the rep that if he wanted his machine he would find it in pieces in the Vanderbilt parking lot — a bit of bravado on my part, but heartfelt nonetheless.

Though I never heard from the rep, my disabling of the soft drink machine stood as a symbol, demonstrating to student athletes and my staff alike the importance of taking food and drink choices seriously – a lesson to be learned by any competitor ready to take a seat at the Training Table.

___ • ___

Chapter 1

Welcome to My Table

The Key to Your Competitive Edge

Show me an athlete whose career is more successful than most and I'll show you a person who is disciplined in all areas of training and diet. Show me recreational athletes who regularly hit the tennis court, golf course, or running track and I'll show you men and women who are among the healthiest and most competitive. If you choose to join their ranks, you'll not only improve your performance but also feel better, have more spring in your step, and may well add years to your life.

Athletes need to eat more frequently than anyone with a sedentary lifestyle – at least 35 times a week, or well over a hundred opportunities a month to enjoy performance-enhancing meals.

Stick to your Training Table program and you'll have a constant supply of carbohydrates, protein, and fat (the three essential macronutrients) and the calories they provide, along with vitamins, minerals, and trace elements (all known as micronutrients). In the short term, you'll also rebalance your intake of carbs, protein, and fat as you approach game day, the bike race, the marathon. In the long run, you'll take a more well-rounded approach to keeping yourself in great shape.

Set Yourself FREE

With all the media attention given to fitness, you're probably aware that a long-term food plan (in place of a few weeks' effort to lose weight and stay fit) is the way to go. And "long-term" describes my week-by-week program for athletes. The athletes I advise happen to be students at Vanderbilt University, but the principles underpinning the program apply to anyone who plays team sports or regularly engages in any other strenuous physical activity.

And just what are those principles? I refer to them with the acronym FREE: Food/Fluids, Rest, Exercise, and Education. A brief overview of each element:

Food/Fluids. Yes, calories do count. But the secret to athlete-friendly meals isn't depriving yourself of the foods you like best; instead, it's calibrating the balance of your carbs/protein/fat intake and watching portion sizes. Then there's hydration. It may surprise you to learn that by the time you feel thirsty, your body is already under-hydrated – the reason you should have at least 8 ounces of fluid eight times a day, whether it comes from the tap, a bottle, a soup bowl, or an orange.

Rest. My Training Table program calls for quiet time as well as exercise (below). Strategic napping also enters the picture, especially when you're unable to get seven or eight hours of sleep nightly.

Exercise. Exercise doesn't have to mean working out at the gym, keeping up with a Zumba video, or doing jumping jacks, abdominal crunches, or push-ups. It can be as easy as walking instead of driving and choosing the stairs over the elevator as you go about your daily routine – and, when convenient, taking brisk half-hour walks.

Education. This amounts to getting a good idea of the nutritive value of each of your weekly meals – that is, the rough number of calories and the grams of carbs, protein, and fat you ingest so you can tailor food choices to your needs. How diligently you crunch the numbers is a matter of choice, but learning which foods are working with you – or against you– is essential. (See also "No Calculator Required!" in Chapter 2, Getting Started.)

--- *Take Note* ---

Farewell to the Food Pyramid

In 2006 the Center for Nutrition Policy and Promotion (CNPP), a branch of the United States Department of Agriculture, went electronic with our long-standing guide to a nutritious diet – the food pyramid – and updated the five basic food groups. Today Choose My Plate (www.choosemyplate.gov) groups food and drink as follows:

- **Grains Group** Whole grains, refined grains
- **Vegetables Group** Dark leafy greens, red and orange vegetables, beans and peas,* starchy vegetables, other vegetables
- **Fruits Group** Tree fruits, vine fruits, berries,100% fruit juice
- **Dairy Group** Milk, milk-based desserts,

calcium-fortified soy milk, cheese, yogurt

- **Protein Foods Group** Meats, poultry, sea-food, eggs, nuts, seeds

Another big difference from days past: Choose My Plate's interactive My Pyramid Food Guidance System (www.mypyramidtracker.gov/planner/) allows you to plan and track your diet online.

*Also included in Protein Foods Group

--- • ---

Training Table Checklist

All in all, developing a Training Table program to fit your needs revolves around the ten steps shown below. Aside from planning your 35 meals a week (that is, 21 "real" meals and 14 snacks), you'll want to exercise and know when to rest your body and mind. (Note: For weight loss–maintenance and weight-gain Training Table prototypes see Chapter 4, Eating Smart.)

1. Establish calories needed on days of in-tense activity and on those with lesser activity. (See "Balancing Calories from Carbs, Protein, and Fat" in Chapter 3, Planning Your Weekly Menus.)

2. Plan your menu of five meals/snacks per day for the coming week.

3. Eat breakfast within 30 minutes of waking up.

4. Eat a nutritionally balanced lunch, even if it means making a sandwich or wrap and taking it to work.

5. Have healthful snacks on hand, not only to satisfy hunger in mid-morning and mid-afternoon but also to keep your metabolism humming.

6. Center your dinner around high-protein foods so your body can better restore itself as you sleep.

7. Exercise for a specified time period at least five times a week. (See Chapter 10, Working Out, Weighing In.)

8. Ingest at least eight 8-ounce glasses of fluid daily, and more to pre-hydrate your body before a game or any other extended period of intense physical activity. (See Chapter 9, Hydration, Hydration, Hydration.)

9. Learn which foods and supplements help prevent, treat, or speed recovery

of sickness, bruises, and aches. (See Chapter 12, Fighting Illness, Healing Injuries.)

10. In the evenings leading up to a competition, keep distractions to a minimum. (See Chapter 11, Rest to Be Your Best.)

Your Five Meals a Day

Naturally, what you eat is at the core of an effective Training Table program, as is making sure you don't skip any of your five daily meals. Moreover, when planning your weekly menu you'll want to look not only at calories, macronutrients, and micronutrients but also foods you find tasty, satisfying, and enjoyable. Note: In some cases, especially when your goal is to bulk up, add a sixth meal: an after dinner or late night snack, as noted in the Weight Gain Training Table Sampler in Chapter 4.

Whether you're an aspiring or seasoned athlete, you may not realize just how dramatically food affects your performance and overall fitness. Consider the following:

- Menus too heavy in *carbohydrates* can lessen your absorption of all the vitamins, minerals, and trace elements critical to general health and slow the repair of damaged muscles and tissues.

- Menus with too much *protein* and *fat* can leave you huffing and puffing during your workouts and underperforming on the field, court, or track.
- Menus lacking in *vitamin D* hamper your body's ability to absorb bone-building calcium, while a deficiency of *B vitamins* keeps you from firing up your metabolism and, in turn, your energy level.

For these reasons and more, food picks for your five daily meals call for forethought. In brief, breakfast and your mid-morning snack are the times to think "high-cal," while for lunch and dinner you should concentrate more on the carbs and protein your menu choices supply.

We'll delve more deeply into meal-by-meal and snack-by-snack choices in Chapter 3, Planning Your Weekly Menus and Chapter 4, Eating Smart – and, as you'll find, it's hardly rocket science. Once you get the hang of keeping "carbs, protein, fat" in mind, choosing the foods that best suit your needs will grow simpler week by week.

Chapter 2

Getting Started

... and Setting Goals

How do you go about creating a Training Table of your own? Begin by taking four steps:

1. Determine your ideal weight. (For team athletes and the keenest "weekend warriors," that can mean your ideal playing weight.)

2. Figure out your metabolic rate.

3. Learn the role of carbohydrates in the diet and determine how large a carb load you should be ingesting.

4. Make sure to remember that a series of thought-out weekly menus will not only improve your athletic performance but also help you stay fit for life.

Gauging Your Body Mass Index

The Body Mass Index (BMI) is seen by many in the sports nutrition community as the most effective tool for gauging body weight and the health risks associated with body fat. The BMI formula involves dividing your weight by your height in inches squared and then multiplying that sum by 703. (For a weight chart based on sex, body frame, and height, see "How Much Should You Weigh?" in Chapter 10, Working Out, Weighing In.)

Translating Your BMI

As you can see here, a difference in seven or eight points in Body Mass Index numbers can move you from "officially" underweight category to the ranks of the overweight.

Body Mass Index	Weight Status
Under 18.5	Underweight
18.5–24.9	Normal
25–29.9	Overweight
30 or over	Obese

If you're lucky, your BMI will lie comfortably in the middle range. Even then, there may be reasons to lose or gain weight, which I delve into in

Chapters 5 and 6. Your doctor may have asked you to lose or gain for general health reasons, or a coach or trainer may have suggested you lose pounds or add muscle mass to make you more competitive.

Finding Your Basal Metabolic Rate (BMR)

In its broadest sense, metabolism defines the cellular chemical reactions that convert various compounds in food into the energy essential for bodily functions. To take charge of your weight and improve performance, figure out 1) your basal metabolic rate (BMR), the amount of calories needed to maintain current weight and get you through an average day; and 2) the ballpark number of calories you need to achieve your athletic goals, and where those calories come from.

A person's daily metabolic rate differs according to age and sex, as these mathematical formulas show:

- If you're a male under age 30, estimate your BMR by multiplying your current weight by 15; if you're over 30, multiply by 12.
- If you're a female under 30, multiply your weight by 13; if you're over 30, multiply by 10.4.

Your BMR number is your bedrock, your foundation. Depending on whether you want to build muscle, increase endurance, or lose weight, you'll use it as your starting point for increasing, maintaining, or decreasing calorie intake.

Calories: Burn, Baby, Burn

Even without exercise, your body is busy burning calories. Breathing burns calories. Reading burns calories. And, much like an 18-wheeler requires more fuel to drive 100 miles than a small car, a person who weighs 250 pounds will require more calories to get through the day than someone who weighs under 200.

For example, if you weigh 130 pounds and run three miles in 40 minutes, you'll burn about 450 calories. If you weigh 200 pounds, the same feat will take considerably more calories – around 700. And if you choose to work out every day instead of twice a week, you'll obviously need more calories per week, and vice versa if you want to cut back on your workouts. (See "Calories from Carbs, Protein, and Fat" on page 14.).

Keeping Track of Carbs

Because carbohydrates (the blanket term for sugar, starch, and cellulose) are the organic compounds your body most easily metabolizes into energy, they should be the source of most of your calories. To determine how many carbs you need for peak performance, keep an accurate log of the foods and beverages you consume, and in what amounts, for at least two weeks. Did your energy drop off in the second set of last Saturday's tennis match? Were you able to play two full rounds of golf one week but were too tired to carry on the following week? The answer could lie in your record of calories-from-carbs consumed.

Your meals vary from day to day, of course, so the longer you keep your food log, the more accurate the data will be. Websites such as www.fitday.com provide diet journals, and even smartphone apps like www.MyFitnessPal.com will calculate your results. Alternatively, keep track of your calories-from-carbs intake in a notebook. To arrive at the number of calories each gram of carbs provides, simply multiply the grams by 4.

How else to find nutrition data? One way is to check the Nutrition Facts (carbs included) on prepackaged foods and beverages, which aren't always precise but will serve your purpose (see "Inexact Nutrition Facts" in Chapter 4, Eating Smart). When it comes to calculating the carbohydrate content of fresh foods, check out the sources listed in "Tallying It Up" in Chapter 3, Planning Your Meals.

Calories from Carbs, Protein, and Fat

Once you have a good idea of the amount of carbohydrates you need for peak performance, you'll be ready to gauge your total caloric needs, including calories from protein and fat. Just divide the combined daily total of calories by the number of days you kept track; the result is your average daily caloric intake – your starting point for establishing an effective Training Table.

Imprint on your brain the calories provided by the three macronutrients:

- 1 gram carbohydrates = 4 calories
- 1 gram protein = 4 calories
- 1 gram fat = 9 calories

Then, after your testing period, proceed as needed:

- If you burned 1,000 calories more each

day than you ingested and your aim is to lose weight, good job!

- If you need to maintain your weight, then increase your caloric intake by 500–1,000 calories each day.
- If you, your trainer, or coach (and possibly your parents and/or physician) agree that you need to gain weight, increase your daily calories from carbs and protein by 500–1,000.

Chapter 3

Planning Your Meals

35 Shots at the Right Stuff

As laid out in the Training Table Checklist in Chapter 1, my program involves more than just food – as Fluids, the other half of the "F" in FREE, shows. But it goes without saying that its most important element is what you put on the table after you've determined both your ideal weight and the number of calories you need to achieve your athletic and fitness goals.

Planning Your Menus

The point of planning your daily menus a week ahead is the view it gives you of the big picture. It's all about bringing your total intake of calories, carbohydrates, fat, and protein into the balance – if not every single day, than surely over the course of a week. Read on to learn what your five daily meals are doing for you.

Breakfast. Making meals work for you starts with breakfast. Even if you're not accustomed to putting something in your empty stomach at dawn's early light, you'll do well to eat within 30 minutes of waking up. And don't even think of skipping breakfast! This kick-start meal not only supplies the vital nutrients that increase your energy and improve your mood but also revs up the metabolism that burns calories throughout the day. What's more, breakfast helps replenish the liver glycogen stores your body used overnight, readying you for the workout or exercise you'll do later.

Mid-morning Snack. Who said you shouldn't eat between meals? A morning snack – of high-calorie foods, no less – is valuable, especially when you want to add mass to your frame. If you anticipate strenuous exertion in the next day or two, mid-morning is also a great time for adding carbs. And, if you need protein, this snack can help you regain lost ground.

Lunch. Like breakfast, a healthful lunch can fall victim to today's ever-more-rushed lifestyles, but the last thing you want to do is succumb to the convenience of the fast food drive-thru. Base your food choices on what you've planned for the rest of the day – heavy-duty or light training, a game, or a nice nap.

Mid-afternoon Snack. For successful athletes, an afternoon snack comes shortly before a workout or exercise, so foods full of both carbs and protein (for example, a piece of fruit and half a sandwich) are the preferred choice. Eating 30 minutes before strenuous physical activity helps build muscle more efficiently. As important, the food will be digested as you exercise and then provide the balance of blood glucose, amino acids, and insulin that begin to rebuild your muscles as soon as you finish your regimen.

Dinner. Foods taking center stage at the dinner table should be protein-rich lean meats and legumes, with dairy products in the supporting role. The body needs amino acids, which are protein's building blocks, to repair any bumps, cuts, bruises, or small muscle tears that might have been sustained during the day – and they do their job all the better as you rest.

Adjust Your Carb/Protein/Fat Ratios

As I explained previously, the second "E" in FREE stands for "education," which means getting a good idea of the calorie, carb, protein, and fat content of the food you slot into your weekly menus and when to adapt their intake to your levels of athletic activity, or lack thereof.

Those All-Important "Whens"

The harder your body works, the more instant fuel it needs. Therefore, a carb-heavy meal before exertion has obvious benefits. Still, for this strategy to be truly effective your heavier-than-usual carb intake should start several days ahead of strenuous athletic activity. Not only is it important to provide your body the proper food types in proper quantities, but doing so at the right time is a critical aspect of my food program. Your ideal timing:

- On a resting (sports-free) day, around 60–65 percent of your calories should come from carbs, 15–20 percent from protein, and 20 percent from fat.

- As you practice or train for an athletic event, you'll want to ramp up your carbs while lowering your fat intake.

- On the day of the event, increase your ingestion of carbs and lower your fat intake even more, as the chart below indicates. (For more information on protein and fat, see Chapter 7, Feeding the Athlete in You.)

Balancing Calories from Carbs, Protein, and Fat

Remember that 1 gram of carbs and protein provide 4 calories each, whereas 1 gram of fat provides more than twice the calories – a total of 9.

Macronutrient	Resting Day	Training Day	Game Day
Carbs	60%	70%	75%
Protein	20%	15%	15%
Fat	20%	15%	10%

Tallying It Up

How do you go about determining calorie and macronutrient content of your food? Read on.

- Check the pertinent nutritional data on the labels of prepackaged foods, which is approximate but still serves your needs (see "Inexact Nutrition Facts" sidebar in Chapter 4, Eating Smart).
- Go online to find nutrition data for fresh meat, chicken, fish, produce, and other

foods lacking nutrition counts. Just key the food or beverage into the search field of any of these websites, all three of which are free:

— United States Department of Agriculture (www.nal.usda.gov/fnic/foodcomp/search)

— Calorie King (www.calorieking.com)

— Carbohydrate Counter (www.carbohydratecounter.org)

Check the table of contents or index of nutrition books to see if they offer the info you seek.

No Calculator Required! If you're the type who just can't find enough uses for your calculator, you'll jump at the chance to tally calorie and macronutrient totals. However, my athletes and I make a point of learning only the approximate carb, protein, and fat content of common foods, then go from there. Only if you're an inveterate number cruncher is there reason to be exact.

Sticklers can make it easy on themselves by recording the data in a notebook or an Excel or Word document. For instance, once you've recorded that a medium-size baked potato with 1 tablespoon butter has about 300 calories – with about 85 percent of the calories from carbs, 2 percent from protein, and

50 percent from fat – this bit of data will always be easily at hand. And remember that websites such as www.MyFitnessPal.com and www.my pyramidtracker.gov/planner will take calculating data out of your hands entirely.

Give It Time

Before telling you how to plan own Training Table in the next chapter, I'll caution you to be patient as you work toward your goals. Remember that your Training Table isn't intended as a quick fix – it's a food program for life. Besides, two months after starting you'll feel so good you won't give much consideration to what your bathroom scales said yesterday. Better still, you should be well on your way to reaching your athletic and physical potential – something that will show not only in your performance but also in your physique.

Food and Drink: Star Players

As explained in Chapter 1, my Training Table program includes exercise and rest components. However, it is naturally centered on your food choices, especially since we're talking 35 meals a week. The advice you'll find in the chapters that follow include how to …

- Be your own food coach and plan a Training Table
- Choose foods wisely without giving up what you like
- Expand your range of foods for the sake of fitness, performance, and endurance
- Relate food and drink to effective exercise
- Use food to help your body stave off illness and heal injuries

As a bonus, you'll find prototypical food choices and how many of them compare with similar foods in terms of calories, carbs, protein and fat – and even three separate lists showing the comparative fat content of pizza toppings, the calories in different cheeses, and the carbohydrate content of beverages. If *Eating to Win* changes the way you look at food – and your eating habits start doing you favors on game days – then you're on your way to gaining the competitive edge.

--- Take Note ---

Case Studies

Many a Vanderbilt athlete I've been lucky enough to work with has gone on to success in professional sports. Among them are Heisman Trophy winner and Tennessee Titans running back **Eddie George** *(see profile in Chapter 11, Rest to Be Your Best); NFL stars* **Jay Cutler, Chris Smith, Jevon Kearse,** *and* **Randall Godfrey;** *Major League Baseball pitchers* **Sonny Gray** *and* **David Price;** *and PGA golfer* **Brandt Snedeker.** *Waiting in the wings are a number of Vanderbilt undergraduates who have already gained the attention of major league recruiters. These and many other Vanderbilt athletes' stories are worth telling, but space dictates limiting them to one: how footballer Cutler went from "too skinny" to "just right":*

When Indiana-born Cutler, now quarterback of the Chicago Bears, arrived on the Vanderbilt campus he was a 6'4" beanpole tipping the scales at 195 pounds. After his senior season as a quarterback (2005), he was a 230-pound first-round draft choice of the Denver Broncos. How did he do it? By taking his food program every bit as seriously as he workouts, practices, and games. This slender standout, his parents, and his coaches agreed that he needed to put considerable mass on his lanky frame if he were to play his best and stay unhurt, and Cutler stuck closely to the Training Table program that he and I designed.

Every day Cutler ate a high-cal breakfast without fail. He carried fruit in his backpack to nibble on between classes. He drank smoothies and shakes (a calorie/protein double whammy). He appreciated the nutritive power of the humble peanut butter and jelly sandwich. He made sure never to skip a meal, whether a three-course dinner or a mid-morning snack. And over the next four years he packed on 35 pounds of muscle and rewrote the Vanderbilt football record book.

--- • ---

For Baby Boomers and Beyond ...

If you're like most people aged 50 or over, you like to think your age won't slow you down when it comes to recreational sports. But you know it's a different story for your metabolism, which begins to slow once we hit 30. For that reason, you may already be altering your diet to stay fit and lean – and if not, it's time to begin.

Perhaps the easiest way to move toward making every calorie work for you is to take some facts to heart, some of which may surprise you:

- Potato chips, fried chicken, rich dairy products, and other fatty foods have more than twice the fat of fruits, vegetables, lean meats, and low-fat dairy products.

- The increasing fragility of your bones means you need at least three servings of dairy products a day, whether in the form of milk, yogurt, or cheese. If you find this too much to bite off, consider taking an over-the-counter calcium supplement.

- Did you know your body doesn't absorb vitamin B12 as easily as it once did? Try one of the multivitamins that provide this essential vitamin in a more absorbable form.

- Increased consumption of fruits and vegetables gives the body some of the additional fluids we all need as we age – so stock your kitchen with cucumbers, melons, lemons, and the like and drink up! (See also "Drinks from Garden, Bush, and Tree" in Chapter 9, Hydration, Hydration, Hydration)

If You're the Parent of a Pre-Teen ...

Like any athlete, children need a steady flow of carbs to restock the glycogen stores in the muscles and liver, protein to provide amino acids to help the body grow and repair, and a little unsaturated fat to help absorb many of the vitamins so critical to their very survival. But how can you tell if children are getting the nutrition they need?

Start by watching their performance. Are they constantly trying to play catch up with the other kids, or can they run up and down the basketball court with the best of them? If your child seems a little sluggish, retrace her steps for the past couple of days. Did carbs comprise at least two-thirds of her intake? Was she at a sleepover party the night before and consumed high-fat pizza and caffeine-containing sodas? Is she not getting enough rest (see sleepover)?

Your physician will be able to tell you if your child isn't getting enough of a particular vitamin or mineral. At the same time, to help ensure that he's getting what he needs on a daily basis, it's fine to supplement what should be a well-balanced diet with an over-the-counter multivitamin formulated for kids.

Chapter 4

Eating Smart

Which Foods Fit Your Needs?

———————————

The food choices in this chapter's Training Table samplers give you ideas for planning your menus, whether your goal is to lose, maintain, or gain weight. Remember, however, that the choices are examples only, since one of the advantages of the FREE approach to fitness is eating foods you like best. So long as you tailor your foods and portion sizes to your carb, protein, and fat intake needs, the sky's the limit!

In some portions of the samplers, the calorie and macronutrient counts are based on equal serving sizes, allowing you to compare carb, protein, and fat content at a glance – e.g., dried apricot vs. fresh apricot, red kidney beans vs. black beans, protein bars vs. trail mix.

However your menus take shape, be sure not to shortchange any of the basic food groups, as outlined in "Farewell to the Food Pyramid" in Chapter 1: vegetables; fruits; grains; high-protein foods like meat, poultry, and seafood; and dairy products. And please take note: If you have no taste for vegetables or fruits, bite the bullet and incorporate at least some of these nutritive-rich, no-cholesterol foods into your diet. It may be easier than you think, as explained in "Learning to Like New Foods" in Chapter 7, Feeding the Athlete in You.

Indulgences vs. Never-Evers

If your appetite is sated throughout the day, you're far less likely to heed the siren call of a double cheeseburger with fries. At the same time, sticking to your Training Table menu doesn't mean you can't indulge yourself from time to time. Just remember that the discipline you need to avoid temptation is akin to the discipline it takes to keep to a workout schedule. Exceptions (and non-exceptions) to the rule:

- May you eat a slice of birthday cake at a party? Of course. What about a hot fudge sundae as a reward for a good game? Yes, if it's not humongous.

- May you make a habit of drinking cola and other sugary soft drinks even once or twice a day? Or wolf down three glazed doughnuts 30 minutes before kickoff? The answer to both is a big NO. (See "Playing Hardball with Soft Drinks" in the Introduction, My Road to the Training Table.)

To put it bluntly, a well-planned Training Table program bans virtually all junk food. If you find yourself in the drive-thru lane more than once every few weeks – or worse, on game day – you not only undermine your health but also reduce the chances of reaching your athletic potential.

--- *Take Note* ---

Boy Foods vs. Girl Foods

In some parts of the athletic world, a battle of the sexes is in full swing. But it's a mental one – the idea that there's such a thing as "boy foods" and "girl foods." Think about it: Is a skinless chicken breast more likely to be found on a male athlete's plate or a female's? And doesn't the same go for tofu versus a slab of pork ribs? As silly as the link between food and gender is, it's out there. Frank, who needs to add more calcium to his diet, is reluctant to try low-fat cottage cheese, just as Sarah tends to choose salmon or tuna over a big juicy steak whenever she wants more protein. So what difference does it make? A big one. Frank is avoiding a dairy product that's one of the best sources of calcium, and Sarah's body needs the iron found in red meat.

Variety is an essential element of an athlete's menu, both for good nutrition and satisfaction with one's day-to-day meals. Accordingly, the notion that certain foods are somehow gender appropriate is one that wise men and women (athletes or not) will discard.

___ • ___

A Weight-Loss Training Table Sampler

As you'll note, these food and beverage suggestions for your five daily meals are interspersed with useful info on fruit juice macronutrients, kiwis, alfalfa sprouts, crackers and chips, and a list of breads (a dozen breads grouped together so you can easily compare their calorie and macronutrient counts). Also note that, as a whole, the food choices are neither low-cal nor fat-free ... All could as easily be part of a weight-gain training table, since it's your total daily intake of calories and that matters.

Breakfast

Here are comparisons of some of the breakfast basics, though any healthful food will effectively kick-start your day. Among your choices …

> **Pork breakfast link sausage** (3/4-oz link) 80 calories • 0.1g carbs • 5g protein • 6.5g total fat

> **Turkey breakfast link sausage** (3/4-oz link) 45 calories • 0.4g carbs • 3g protein • 3g total fat

> **Soy breakfast link sausage** (3/4-oz link) 85 calories • 4g carbs • 10g protein • 3g total fat

> **Scrambled eggs** (3 large eggs) 250 calories • 2g carbs • 18.5g protein • 18g total fat

> **Scrambled egg whites** (whites of 3 large eggs) 65 calories • 1g carbs • 14g protein • 0.5g total fat

> **Plain pancake** (6-in. diameter cake, or 2.7 oz, with 2 tsp butter) 160 calories • 16g carbs • 2g protein • 9.5g total fat

Whole wheat pancake (6-in. diameter cake, or 2.7 oz, with 2 tsp butter) 180 calories • 14g carbs • 4g protein • 12.5g total fat

Oatmeal (3/4 cup, plain) 165 calories • 28.5g carbs • 6g protein • 3g total fat

Corn flakes (1/2 cup cereal, 1/4 cup 2% milk) 130 calories • 27g carbs • 4g protein • 3g total fat

Granola (1/2 cup fruit-and-nut granola,1/4 cup 2% milk) 385 calories • 65g carbs • 10g protein • 9g total fat

Orange juice (8 oz) 110 calories; 25g carbs; 1.25g protein; 0.15g total fat

Tomato juice (8 oz) 40 calories; 10g carbs; 2g protein; 0.2g total fat

--- *Take Note* ---

Fruit Juice: The Real Thing?

Unless you squeeze your own fruit juice every morning, it pays to learn how to tell real store-bought juices from not-so-real ones. The "100% juice" claim on labels is allowable only if the product is either pure juice or juice made from concentrates (in the latter case, without added sugars and the like). For this reason, always check the ingredients, which are listed in order of amount.

Case in point: Many blended juices have more filtered water than concentrates – so while the juice may qualify as real, blended juices may have slightly less taste than their no-concentrate counterparts.

How to spot products that don't rise to the real juice level, many with as little as 10% fruit juice? Give-away words include drink, beverage, punch, ade, *and* cocktail. *The larger part of such drinks is generally made up of water, added sugars (often the notorious high fructose corn syrup), and preservatives.*

--- • ---

Mid-Morning Snack

Eating hi-cal foods between breakfast and lunch will fuel you even more, so when you reach for fruits go for apples or bananas or dried fruit (dried fruit is way more calorific than fresh). Yogurt's good too, whether flavored or plain. Among your choices …

> **Bagel with cream cheese** (4-in. diameter bagel with 1.5 Tbsp cheese) 310 calories • 46g carbs • 10g protein • 7.5g total fat

> **Regular yogurt** (8 oz low-fat, plain) 150 calories • 16.5g carbs • 12g protein • 4g total fat

Greek yogurt (8 oz low-fat, plain) 175 calories • 9.5g carbs • 22g protein • 3.5g total fat

Apple (4 oz, or 1 small fruit, unpeeled) 70 calories • 15.5g carbs • 0.5g protein • 0.5g total fat

Banana (4 oz, or one 7-in. long fruit, peeled) 115 calories • 26g carbs • 1.5g protein • 0.5g total fat

Kiwis (4 oz, or 2 small fruits, peeled) 80 calories • 17g carbs • 1.5g protein • 0.5g total fat

Apricots (4 oz, or 3-4 fruits, unpeeled) 65 calories • 13 carbs • 1g protein • 02g total fat

Dried apricots (4 oz, or about ½ cup) 305 calories • 73.5g carbs • 3g protein • 0g total fat

Dried cranberries (4 oz, or about ½ cup, sweetened) 345 calories • 23g carbs • 0g protein • 0.25g total fat

Raisins (4 oz seedless, or about ½ cup) 380 calories • 90g carbs • 3.5g protein • 0.5g total fat

--- *Take Note* ---

An Athlete's Fuzzy Friend

The kiwi is a nutritious fruit formerly known as the Chinese gooseberry. In the 1970s, it was New Zealanders who dubbed it kiwi fruit and cornered the market on its cultivation. For a zesty treat, either slice through the fuzzy skin and scoop out the green pulp or peel and slice the fruit.

Kiwi is a great source of both potassium and vitamin C, which for athletes is all the more valuable because C strengthens blood vessel walls and promotes the absorption of endurance-building ferrous sulfate, better known as iron.

--- • ---

Lunch

Time to steer clear of the fast food outlet! But that doesn't mean you can't indulge yourself at midday. The trick is to balance the intake of calories in your weekly menu, and paying particular attention to carbs at lunchtime. Among your choices …

> **Franks and beans** (1 cup sliced beef frankfurter, canned baked beans, onion, brown sugar, mustard) 350 calories • 54g carbs • 8g protein • 10g total fat

Caesar salad with grilled chicken (7.5 oz salad, 2 oz chicken breast) 200 calories • 9g carbs • 22.5g protein • 7.5 total fat

Turkey-alfalfa tortilla wrap (6-in. diameter flour tortilla with sliced turkey, alfalfa sprouts, grated carrot, grated cheese) 225 calories • 18g carbs • 14g protein • 10g total fat

Garlic shrimp and angel hair pasta (1 cup pasta, shrimp, garlic, olive oil, Parmesan cheese) 300 calories • 33g carbs • 24g protein • 7.5g total fat

Spicy tuna California roll (3 pieces) 150 calories • 18g carbs • 7.5g protein • 4g total fat

Spaghetti Bolognese (2/3 cup pasta, 1/3 cup tomato sauce with pork and beef) 150 calories • 27g carbs • 5g protein • 2g total fat

Spaghetti Alfredo (2/3 cup pasta, 1/3 cup cream sauce with egg and Parmesan cheese) 210 calories • 23g carbs • 6g protein • 11g total fat

Veggie burger patty (3 oz, pan-fried) 160 calories • 12g carbs • 16g protein • 5g total fat

Asparagus (3 oz, or about 4 medium-thick spears) 24 calories • 2.5g carbs • 1.5g protein • 0.15g total fat

Green peas (3 oz) 75 calories • 13g carbs • 4.5g protein • 0.3g total fat

Sugar snap peas (3 oz) 40 calories • 6g carbs • 2.5g protein • 0.3g total fat

Bell pepper (1/2 cup, chopped) 24 calories • 5.2g carbs • 0.8g protein • 0.5g total fat

Whole kernel corn (1/2 cup canned, drained) 65 calories • 15g carbs • 2g protein • 1g total fat

Pickled beets (1/2 cup sliced, drained) 80 calories • 18g carbs • 1g protein • 6g total fat

Pineapple with cottage cheese (2 canned slices, drained; 2 Tbsp 4% fat cottage cheese) 70 calories • 27g carbs • 6.25g protein • 1g total fat

Pineapple with grated cheese (2 canned slices, drained; 2 Tbsp grated cheddar) 150 calories • 12g carbs • 3g protein • 9.5g total fat

--- *Take Note* ---

Fill 'er Up with Alfalfa

To pack a lot of nutrition (but very few calories) into sandwiches and salads, add raw alfalfa sprouts. Alfalfa is

rich in dietary fiber and protein, and it's a terrific source of vitamins A, C, and K – not to mention a lengthy list of other good stuff, like niacin, calcium, thiamin, riboflavin, folate, pantothenic acid, iron, magnesium, phosphorus, zinc, copper, and manganese. Who would have guessed that so much nutrition could be crammed into such a humble plant? What's more, it adds a nice crunch to meals.

Do be careful, though. From 1997 to 2002, salmonella outbreaks in alfalfa crops led to sickness in consumers in several states. Guard against illness by making sure you 1) buy spouts and other fresh vegetables at a food store known for the care it takes with produce, and 2) thoroughly rinse produce of any kind before storing it in the fridge.

___ • ___

Mid-Afternoon Snacks

For many of us, an afternoon snack comes shortly before a workout or exercise, making foods full of both carbs and protein the preferred picks. Among your choices …

> **Pita chips and hummus** (1 oz chips, or about 6, plus 2 Tbsp hummus) 185 calories • 23g carbs • 5g protein • 8g total fat

Carrot slices and onion dip (2.5 oz raw carrots, 1.5 tbsp dip) 75 calories • 8.5g carbs • 2g protein • 3.5g total fat

Broccoli florets and onion dip (2.5 oz raw broccoli, 1.5 tbsp dip) 68 calories • 6.5g carbs • 2g protein • 3.5g total fat

Oil-popped popped corn (4 oz) 55 calories • 6.5g carbs • 1g protein • 3g total fat

Air-popped popcorn (4 oz) 15 calories • 3g carbs • 0.5g protein • 0.5g total fat

Strawberries with yogurt (1/2 plain low-fat yogurt, 6 medium-size strawberries) 120 calories • 14g carbs • 6.5g protein • 4g total fat

Mango (4 oz raw, sliced) 80 calories • 20g carbs • 0g protein • 0g total fat

Papaya (4 oz raw, sliced) 50 calories • 12g carbs • 0g protein • 0g total fat

Grapes (4 oz white or red, or about 24 grapes) 90 calories • 9g carbs • 1g protein • 0.5g total fat

Watermelon (4-oz wedge) 45 calories • 13g carbs • 1g protein • 0.3g total fat

--- *Take Note* ---

Crackers, Chips, Et Cetera

Wondering how the pita chips used to scoop up hummus and other dips fare in the carbs and fat stakes? A 3½-ounce serving of chips only has about 20 carbs and 5 grams total fat. But how do other dippers compare? When you have the same 3½-ounce serving without dip, like this:

- Heading the eating-to-win class are matzo (84g carbs, 5g fat); melba toast (77g carbs, 1.5g fat); and rye crispbread (82g carbs and 1.5g fat; and plain pita bread (55g and 2.5g respectively).

- At the back of the class are ordinary potato chips (50g carbs and 38g fat)–and the baked potato chips (71g carbs and 18g fat) are a little better, but not that much.

- In mid-range are tortilla chips, with regular chips coming in at 66g carbs and 23g fat, and baked tortilla chips registering 80g and 6g respectively.

The dippers with the most protein? Melba toast, baked tortilla chips, and matzo, all with 10 to 12 grams. The lowest?

Again, potato chips of any sort, all with about half the protein of the champs.

--- • ---

Dinner

If you're trying to lose weight, go for the lo-cal, lo-fat version of a favorite food as your main course of the day; in the meat and poultry department, that means turkey chili over beef chili and roasted chicken over fried. On quiet nights at home, think beyond food choice and enhance meals by "resting to be your best," as discussed in Chapter 11. Among your choices ...

> **Beef flank steak** (4 oz. grilled) 180 calories • 0g carbs • 28g protein • 7g total fat
>
> **Pork tenderloin** (4 oz, roasted) 135 calories • 0.35g carbs • 24g protein • 4g total fat
>
> **Beef chili** (1 cup with red kidney beans, tomatoes, onions, green chiles) 400 calories • 10g carbs • 26g protein • 9g total fat
>
> **Turkey chili** (1 cup with red kidney beans, tomatoes, onions, green chiles) 240 calories • 30g carbs • 19g protein • 4.5g total fat

Fried chicken (3-oz breast, skinned and boned) 210 calories • 0.6g carbs • 38.5g protein • 5.25g total fat

Roast chicken (3-oz breast, skinned and boned) 185 calories • 0g carbs • 37.5g protein • 4g total fat

Ground pork patty (4 oz, pan-fried) 285 calories • 0g carbs • 4g protein • 24g total fat

Ground turkey patty (4 oz, pan-fried) 285 calories • 0g carbs • 30g protein • 18g total fat

Salmon (4 oz. grilled) 160 calories • 0g carbs • 21g protein • 3.25g total fat

Halibut (4 oz baked) 125 calories • 0g carbs • 25.5g protein • 2g total fat

Endamame salad (2 cups with shelled green soybeans, romaine lettuce, pickled beets, grated ginger, sesame oil-soy sauce dressing) 260 calories • 40g carbs • 26g protein • 10g total fat

Cherry tomato salad (2 cups with cucumber, green onion, Italian dressing) 125 calories • 14g carbs • 3.5g protein • 6g total fat

Broccoli (4 oz, steamed) 30 calories • 6g carbs • 2g protein • 0.3g total fat

Kale (4 oz, steamed) 24 calories • 5g carbs • 1.5g protein • 0.3g total fat

Corn on the cob (1 medium-size ear) 60 calories • 14g carbs • 2g protein • 0.5g total fat

Buttered corn on the cob (1 medium-size ear with ½ Tbsp butter) 110 calories • 14g carbs • 2g protein • 6g total fat

Loaded baked potato (1 large, or 10 oz, with skin, butter, sour cream, grated cheddar, bacon bits) 680 calories • 70g carbs • 14g protein • 10g total fat

Low-fat baked potato (1 large, or 10 oz, with skin, butter substitute, and seasoned salt) 350 calories • 60g carbs • 9g protein • 0g total fat

Sweet potato (4 oz, with skin) 105 calories • 24g carbs • 2.25g protein • 0.25g total fat

––– Take Note –––

1 Ounce Bread = ??

Bread competes with pasta as the carb lover's best friend. And though white bread has the edge over whole grain breads when it comes to carbs, its re-fined wheat flour isn't as good for you overall.

Reminder: Calorie and macronutrient counts are based on a 1-ounce slice or wedge.

Bagel, Plain 85 calories • 15g carbs • 3g protein • 1.5g total fat

Corn Bread 140 calories • 23g carbs • 4.5g protein • 8g total fat

Crispbread 10 calories • 14g carbs • 2g protein • 0g total fat

Multigrain* 75 calories • 12g carbs • 4g protein • 1g total fat

Naan 70 calories • 11g carbs • 3g protein • 1g total fat

Pita 75 calories • 16g carbs • 3g protein • 0g total fat

Pizza Crust 100 calories • 18g carbs • 4.5g protein • 2g total fat

Pumpernickel 70 calories • 13g carbs • 2g protein • 1g total fat

Rye 65 calories • 12.5g carbs • 2.5g protein • 1g total fat

Sourdough 85 calories • 15.5g carbs • 3g protein • 1g total fat

White 100 calories • 20g carbs • 3g protein • 0g total fat

Whole wheat 65 calories • 12g carbs • 4g protein • 1g total fat

* Grains vary from brand to brand.

___ • ___

Every day of the week ...

- Keep healthful snacks readily available.

- Don't skip meals or snacks; instead, make them smaller.

- Be sure you take in 60 to 70 fluid ounces of fluid, whether from a glass or bottle or from food.

- Make room daily for at least one 20 to 60 minute exercise session.

- Refrain from eating two hours before bedtime.

Inexact Nutrition Facts

The Food & Drug Administration (FDA) requires food and beverage manufacturers to put Nutrition Facts on their labels, starting with calories per serving and progressing to grams of total fat, carbohydrates, and protein and the daily value amount of selected vitamins and minerals. The fact is, the numbers are rarely precise. And why is this so? Largely because …

- The output of most manufacturers varies slightly from batch to batch, so it only makes sense for calorie and gram counts on labels to be ballpark estimates.

- The FDA gives manufacturers a good deal of leeway by allowing a 20 percent margin of error.

- It is legal for grams to be rounded off to the nearest fifth in some cases, and to the nearest tenth in others.

In the nutrition data appearing in *Eating to Win*, calorie counts are "corrected" by adding up the number of calories from carbs (4), protein (4), and total fat (9) – and, as a result, the calories cited in the weight loss–maintenance and weight gain charts in this chapter won't always jibe with those on the label of brand name products. Nor is there any guarantee that the macronutrient counts on labels are exact, but this book's data comparisons of one food choice to another remain solid.

A Weight-Gain Training Table Sampler

Ah, chili … grilled cheese sandwiches … muffins! If you're trying to gain weight, you can pretty much throw caution to the winds. At the same time, make sure the calories you take in come more from carbs than from fat, lest you gain flab instead of muscle. You also have room for a sixth meal every day: the late-night snack, six examples of which are offered at the end of this chart.

Breakfast

No need to say "hold the bacon" to the household cook or the restaurant server. Nor do you need to eat reduced-fat cereals or watch the calories in fruit juice so long as you keep your weekly menus on the right track. Among your choices …

> **Bacon** (2 slices fried, or about 3/4 oz) 95 calories • 0.1g carbs • 6g protein • 7g total fat

> **Soy breakfast patties** (2 patties, or 2.5 oz) 160 calories • 6g carbs • 20g protein • 6g total fat

> **Cheese and tomato omelet** (3 large eggs, ½ cup Cheddar cheese, ¼ cup diced tomato) 425 calories • 3g carbs • 28g protein • 33g total fat

Fried eggs (2, fried in canola or safflower oil) 175 calories • 0g carbs • 12g protein • 14g total fat'

Eggs Benedict (poached egg, Canadian bacon, ½ English muffin, Hollandaise sauce) 410 calories • 15g carbs • 14g protein • 33g total fat

Waffle (6-in. diameter plain, with 2 tsp butter and 1 Tbsp maple syrup) 275 calories • 37g carbs • 4g protein • 8g total fat

French toast (1 thick bread slice, or 3 oz, with 1 Tbsp maple syrup) 255 calories • 46g carbs • 12g protein • 1g total fat

Cream of wheat (1 cup, cooked) 155 calories • 32g carbs • 4g protein • 1g total fat

Muesli (1 cup cereal, ½ cup 2% milk) 370 calories • 66g carbs • 12g protein • 6g total fat

Cranberry juice (8 oz) 120 calories; 30g carbs; 1g protein; 1g total fat

Pomegranate juice (8 oz) 145 calories; 36g carbs; 0g protein; 0g total fat

Fruit smoothie (8 oz vanilla yogurt blended with 2 oz raspberries, 2 oz blueberries) 290 calories • 53g carbs • 11g protein • 3g total fat

––– Take Note –––

Go, Yogurt, Go!

Yogurt is worth cheering for. It not only makes a good base for a tasty milkshake but also works as a substitute for sour cream or mayo in homemade dips and salad dressings. On the health front, yogurt increases the amount of calcium in your diet while cutting calories. Another plus is that this fermented milk's bacterial cultures – especially those from the bacterium Lactobacillus acidophilus – help keep your gastrointestinal system in good working order.

––– • –––

Mid-Morning Snack

You can easily afford a milkshake or smoothie between breakfast and lunch, and you can take a cue from some of the eager-to-bulk-up athletes I advise and add cashews or peanuts to the blender. Having your shake while munching on dried fruit or a whole grain muffin will really help you put on pounds. Among your choices …

Fresh figs (2 oz) 50 calories • 11g carbs • .05g protein • 0.2g total fat

Dried figs (2 oz) 150 calories • 35g carbs • 0.25g protein • 0.5g total fat

Fig Newtons (2 oz, or 3 bars) 165 calories • 33g carbs • 1.5g protein • 3g total fat

Corn muffin (4 oz) 485 calories • 58g carbs • 7g protein • 22g total fat

Raisin bran muffin (4 oz) 435 calories • 80g carbs • 4.5g protein • 10.5g total fat

Blueberry muffin (4 oz) 400 calories • 50g carbs • 6.5g protein • 19g total fat

Dry-roasted soynuts (2 oz, or ¼ cup) 270 calories • 18g carbs • 22g protein • 12g total fat

Graham crackers (0.85 oz, or six 2 ½ - sq. in. crackers) 200 calories • 36g carbs • 12g protein • 5g total fat

Vanilla milkshake (8 oz; 1/3 cup whole milk, 1 cup ice cream, packed) 450 calories • 48g carbs • 10g protein • 24g total fat

Carnation Instant Breakfast® (1 packet in 8 oz fat-free milk) 220 calories • 9g carbs • 5g protein • 0g total fat

––– *Take Note* –––

Let's Hear It for Fruit!

Keeping a basketful of fruit out in the open will ensure that healthy foods are readily available when snack

attacks sneak up on you. For variety, branch out beyond apples, oranges, bananas, pears, plums, and strawberries. Tropical fruits like mango, papaya, guava, and lychee will keep you from tiring of the same-old, same-old.

––– • –––

Lunch

If you're a dedicated athlete, you may or may not be partial to light lunches – but if you are, make sure not to get in a rut and have the salads entrées (typically with grilled chicken or salmon) each day. Variety is not only the spice of life but also is key to good nutrition. Among your choices …

Taco salad (Taco bowl with seasoned ground beef, lettuce, tomato, sour cream, grated cheddar) 580 calories • 74g carbs • 26g protein • 42g total fat

Chinese spring rolls (6 oz, or 2 rolls, with pork, dried mushroom, bell pepper, bean sprouts, oyster sauce) 400 calories • 40g carbs • 24g protein • 12g total fat

Grilled ham and cheese sandwich (rye bread, Gruyère cheese, ham slice, spicy brown mustard) 295 calories • 27g carbs • 7.5g protein • 13g total fat

Chicken, almond, and vegetable stir-fry (chicken breast strips, almonds, carrots, green beans, chicken broth, soy sauce, sesame oil) 390 calories • 20g carbs • 32g protein • 20g total fat

Red pizza (7-in. diameter crust with mozzarella and red meat sauce) 535 calories • 67g carbs • 31g protein • 31g total fat

White pizza (7-in. diameter crust with Alfredo sauce, mozzarella, ricotta, spinach, garlic) 765 calories • 63g carbs • 23g protein • 45g total fat

Fettuccine with smoked salmon (1 cup spinach pasta, smoked salmon, cream sauce of half-and-half, dill, Parmesan cheese) 145 calories • 17g carbs • 5.5g protein • 5g total fat

Tuna salad-stuffed avocado (peeled avocado half, 1/3 cup tuna salad) 375 calories • 16g carbs • 9g protein • 30g total fat

Falafel sandwich (half a 7-in. diameter pita pocket with falafel, lettuce, tomato, tahini sauce) 510 calories • 72g carbs • 20g protein • 17g total fat

Potato salad (1 cup cubed potatoes with celery, onion, parsley, boiled egg, mayonnaise) 330 calories • 28g carbs • 7g protein • 0g total fat

Carrot and raisin salad (1 cup grated carrot, 1 Tbsp raisins, 1.5 tsps ranch dressing) 135 calories • 22g carbs • 1.5g protein • 4g total fat

Bow-tie pasta salad (1 cup pasta with diced tomato, green olives, Italian dressing) 245 calories • 38g carbs • 9g protein • 10g total fat

Sweet 'n' sour red cabbage (I cup cooked cabbage with onion, cider vinegar, brown sugar, butter) 85 calories • 15g carbs • 4g protein • 4g total fat

Tofu-stuffed mushrooms (2 medium-size white mushrooms with tofu, green onion, garlic, oyster sauce, soy sauce) 230 calories • 33g carbs 13g protein • 5g total fat

Macaroni and cheese (4 oz) 230 calories • 24g carbs • 10g protein • 12g total fat

Cous cous (4 oz, cooked) 90 calories • 18g carbs • 4g protein • 0g total fat

--- *Take Note* ---

A Healthful Add-On

When you want to gain weight or add complex carbs to your Training Table menu, have a small side dish of whole-wheat pasta (about a cup, cooked) with each meal

or as a lunch or dinner follow-up. Stirring in a little olive oil or no-trans fats margarine will add more flavor and keep your snack on the healthful side.

--- • ---

Mid-Afternoon Snack

Carb-rich foods like dried fruit, fig bars, date bars, and granola bars will give your body the instant fuel it needs both during and after weight lifting or exercise. On the practical side, no-fuss snacks such as these are easy to carry in a backpack or bag. Among your choices …

> **Peanut butter and jelly sandwich** (2 slices whole wheat bread, 1.5 Tbsp each peanut butter and grape jelly) 355 calories • 32g carbs • 25g protein • 14g total fat

> **Swiss cheese and crackers** (1 Tbsp grated cheese, 6 saltines) 160 calories • 14g carbs • 7.5 protein • 8g total fat

> **Feta-walnut dip and crackers** (1/2 cup dip of feta cheese, yogurt, chopped walnut, and minced garlic with ½-oz water crackers, or about 5) 330 calories • 18g carbs 13.5g protein • 22g fat

Guacamole and tortilla chips (1/2 cup dip with 1 oz chips, or about 10) 345 calories • 27g carbs • 6g protein • 23g fat

Medjool dates (2.5 oz, or 3 dates) 195 calories • 72g carbs • 0g protein • 0g total fat

Generic protein bar (2.5 oz) 280 calories • 30g carbs • 23g protein • 7g total fat

Generic granola bar (2.5 oz) 270 calories • 18g carbs • 10g protein • 6g total fat

Generic trail mix (2.5 oz) 340 calories • 30g carbs • 19g protein • 15g total fat

Raw flax cookies (2.5 oz, or 4 cookies) 300 calories • 17g carbs • 20g protein • 14g total fat

Strawberry-banana smoothie (4 oz each whole milk and vanilla ice cream blended with 2 oz each strawberry and banana) 520 calories • 80g carbs • 17.5g protein • 15g total fat

--- *Take Note* ---

1 Ounce Nuts = ??

Nuts may be high in fat, but more important to athletes is their hefty protein content – though some, as you'll see below, have more carbs than protein. In any case, nuts are an excellent choice during your two snacking periods each day. Reminder: Calorie and macronutrient counts are based on 1 ounce of raw nuts.

Almond 185 calories • 5.5g carbs • 6g protein • 14g total fat

Brazil nut 200 calories • 3g carbs • 4g protein • 19g total fat

Cashew 170 calories • 8.5g carbs • 5g protein • 12g total fat

Hazelnut 190 calories • 5g carbs • 4g protein • 17g total fat

Macadamia 255 calories • 14g carbs • 2g protein • 21g total fat

Peanut 185 calories • 4g carbs • 8g protein • 15g total fat

Pecan 200 calories • 4g carbs • 2.5g protein • 20g total fat

Pistachio 170 calories • 8g carbs • 5g protein • 12.5g total fat

Walnut 195 calories • 4g carbs • 4.5g protein • 18.5 total fat

___ • ___

Dinner

Red meat, white meat, or fish are the high-protein basis for most evening meals, and cheese dishes are protein-rich as well. So are the legumes we call beans, and in this chart you'll find comparisons of the calorie and macronutrient counts of several kinds of this menu staple. Among your choices …

Braised pork chops (4 oz, or 1 bone-in chop, dredged in seasoned flour and braised in chicken broth) 240 calories • 0.5g carbs • 8.5g protein • 2g total fat

Beef and green bean stir-fry (4 oz; flank steak, green beans, onion, garlic, beef broth) 255 calories • 10g carbs • 20g protein • 17g total fat

Tuna steak (4 oz, pan-fired) 125 calories • 0g carbs • 28g protein • 1g total fat

Linguine with white clam sauce (4 oz) 150 calories • 13g carbs • 6.5g protein • 7g total fat

Spinach soufflé (4 oz; egg, spinach, cheddar, milk, butter) 295 calories • 6g carbs • 20.5g protein • 20g total fat

Chiles rellenos (4 oz; cheese-egg mixture in Poblano peppers) 225 calories • 10g carbs • 20g protein • 37g total fat

Cheese grits (1/2 cup cooked grits, ¼ cup grated cheddar) 145 calories • 11.5g carbs • 6g protein • 1g total fat

Creamed spinach (1 cup spinach with whole milk, light cream, butter, garlic) 240 calories • 13g carbs • 20g protein • 18g total fat

Mashed potatoes (1 cup, with 2 oz whole milk, 1.5 tsp butter) 245 calories • 36g carbs • 4g protein • 9g total fat

Mashed butternut squash (1 cup, with 2 oz whole milk, 1.5 tsp butter) 215 calories • 28g carbs • 5g protein • 9g total fat

Curried chickpeas (1 cup peas with diced onion, cilantro, curry powder) 300 calories • 55g carbs • 13g protein • 3g fat

Black-eyed peas (1 cup canned) 195 calories • 32g carbs • 12g protein • 1g total fat

Black beans (1 cup canned) 200 calories • 34g carbs • 12g protein • 1g total fat

Red kidney beans (1 cup canned) 235 calories • 40g carbs • 16g protein • 1g total fat

Lentils (1 cup canned) 240 calories • 42g carbs • 16g protein • 0.5g total fat

Pinto beans (1 cup canned) 250 calories • 45g carbs • 15g protein • 2.5g total fat

White rice (1/2 cup cooked, with olive oil, onion, chicken broth) 105 calories • 23g carbs • 2g protein • 0.25g total fat

Brown rice pilaf (1/2 cup cooked, with olive oil, onion, chicken broth) 125 calories • 23g carbs • 2.5g protein • 0.5g total fat

Spanish rice (1/2 cup, cooked with tomato juice, onion, green bell pepper) 110 calories • 20g carbs • 2.5g protein • 2g total fat

––– *Take Note* –––

A Lift from Legumes

Legumes –which include kidney beans, pinto beans, lima beans, black-eyed peas, and lentils – are an outstanding source of protein, a component critical to building muscle and making repairs to damaged tissues and organs. Plus, beans provide the vital nutrient iron, which helps your circulatory system deliver performance-enhancing oxygen to your muscles during a game.

––– • –––

Late-Night Snack (Optional)

As long as you don't stuff yourself, go ahead and have that midnight snack when you're trying to put on pounds. When else can you raid the fridge or the cookie jar without a guilty conscience? Among your choices ...

Turkey meatloaf (4-oz slice, cold) 180 calories • 0g carbs • 22g protein • 8g total fat

Apple pie (1 slice) 340 calories • 42g carbs • 2g protein • 18g total fat

Warm milk with Ovaltine® (8 oz whole milk, 1 Tbsp Classic Malt Ovaltine) 175 calories • 17.5g carbs • 8g protein • 8g total fat

Chocolate chip cookies (40g, or 3 cookies) 180 calories • 27g carbs • 1.5g protein • 7.5g total fat

Oatmeal raisin cookies (40g, or 2 cookies) 160 calories • 24g carbs • 2g protein • 7g total fat

Ginger snaps (40g, or 5 cookies) 145 calories • 28g carbs • 1.25g protein • 3g total fat

Every Day of the Week ...

- Drink 2% milk instead of 1% or skim/fat-free milk. Choose whole milk only if your saturated fat intake from other sources (e.g., fatty meats, butter) is low.

- When eating high-calorie foods, go for the most nutritious. For instance, choose brown rice over white rice and peanut butter or a soy milkshake over glazed doughnuts or candy.

- Eat high-protein foods that build muscle mass, such as tuna, buckwheat noodles, lean ground beef, turkey breast, and cottage cheese.

- Add extra complex carbs to your diet by eating plenty of vegetables and whole-grain pastas, breads, and cereals.

- At least four times a week, do an hour of muscle-building resistance exercise to help muscles store more energy-producing glycogen.

Chapter 5

Your Weight-Loss Training Table

Getting it Off, Keeping it Off

If you've found it hard to lose pounds, don't fret. Unlike some other approaches to weight loss, my program isn't about depriving yourself of food. Instead, it provides your body with the food it needs 1) in the proper quantities and 2) at the most opportune time. Better still, the effects are long-term – life-long, in fact, if you stick with it.

How Much Should You Lose?

For an athlete of any kind, the decision of how much weight to lose is best made in consultation with your physician, trainer, coach, or all of the above. Their input will help ensure that your target weight is practical, safe, and improves your athletic activity. These "consultants" will also help you establish a reasonable timetable for arriving at your target weight. (See also Chapter 2, Getting Started.)

As numerous studies have shown, Americans on the whole are heavier than ever, with high-fat diets, king-sized portions, and sedentary lifestyles largely responsible. In contrast to competitive athletes, whom coaches urge to lose weight to improve performance on the field or court, average Americans should slim down mainly for health reasons. "Average Americans" includes recreational athletes, of course, who should take that bit of advice to heart: Staying relatively trim and fit will help improve your tennis or golf game or speed your sprint to the finish line. As a soccer coach I knew would say, "The difference between 'fit' and 'fat' is just one letter. But it's a big letter."

Balanced Eats

Does cutting calories mean exiling yourself to a world of bland lunches, dinners, and snacks? Certainly not. You can dine like the choosiest gourmet so long as you 1) take in the proper balance of calories from carbs, protein, and fat; 2) continue to exercise; and 3) bring your calories and balance of macronutrients into line by adjusting your portion sizes – the key to making the foods you'll be eating 35 times each week work for you.

Patience, Please!

Patience is the first thing I stress to an athlete whose goal is to lose weight. Sure, you can drop a couple of pounds in a day by sweating and not replacing lost fluids. And you can shed pounds at a pretty amazing rate with some fad diets. But as a health-conscience person, you should never forget that rapidly achieved results are rarely results that last.

Measuring Up. To gauge weight loss, measure your waistline with a tape measure instead of stepping on the bathroom scales. Why? Because when your body fat is being replaced by muscle mass, your weight may well stay the same, or even increase. You know you're losing body fat when your clothing sizes go down, your blood circulation improves, and your body shape changes – all better indicators that you're shaping up than just keeping track of your poundage.

––– Take Note –––

I've Been There

One big benefit of dropping pounds is the decreased wear and tear on your feet, knees, and back – all common complaints of people who are overweight. Imagine walking along without a care in the world, smiling as you watch the scenery and waving to those you pass by. Now imagine walking the same route with a 25-pound bag of sand hung around your waist. Rather than smiling and waving, you'll probably be thinking about how sore your body is from head to toe and how hard it is to catch your breath.

I know what it's like to be overweight because I've been there, having once carried 20 more pounds than I do today. And how does it feel to lose take it off and keep it off? In a word, great! My joints no longer hurt, and going for a bike ride with my daughter is once again a joy, not a burden. I'm a 50-something "weekend warrior," and I love it.

––– • –––

Maintaining Weight Loss

When a Training Table program does its job, athletes spend most of their time working to maintain their weight – i.e., the weight at which they perform most effectively. If keeping weight from fluctuating is your goal, your M.O. obviously involves burning the same number of calories you take in, be it 1,500 or 3,000. A 500-calorie-per-day imbalance on either side will change your weight by one pound gained or lost each week.

Keep in mind that there's no finish line when it comes to weight management, an idea that ensnares many dieters and dooms them to bounce back to their original weight in a hurry. Whether your doctor or trainer (or you yourself) has determined that you need to lose 8 pounds for performance enhancement or 20 pounds for health reasons, it's essential to maintain your target weight over the months and years.

The Training Table Advantage. We all know that old habits die hard, which is precisely why dieting so often fails. Many people view dieting as a means to an end, the "means" being routine deprivation. Others have no intention of continuing the diet once the desired weight is reached, at which point they revert to their old habits.

Your Training Table diet differs in that it's not about deprivation. Once you've achieved your preferred weight, gradually alter your snacks and meals to stabilize it. If calorie restriction is your goal, for instance, then incorporate additional calories to your Training Table to match the number of calories you expect to burn each day.

The Theory of Relativity. One complicating factor is what I call "the theory of relativity." It has nothing to do with Einstein but everything to do with watching what others eat and jumping to conclusions about your own needs. For instance, you arrive at a cafeteria and notice that skinniest person in line is loading up on high-calorie French fries. You ask yourself, "If she stays that skinny while eating so many fries, why can't I?" Well, for all you know, the svelte customer saved room in her day's caloric intake for just such an indulgence. And even then, you might have caught her on the once-in-a-blue-moon day she gives in to temptation.

Daily Calories for Maintaining Weight

As we age, metabolism slows and we need slightly fewer calories – and just how many depends on our age, gender, height and weight. Two cases in point:

- A moderately active 25-year-old man who weighs 180 and is 6 feet tall needs roughly 2,850 calories each day to maintain his weight. A 45-year-old man of the same weight and height needs about 2,700 daily calories to keep weight steady.

• A moderately active 25-year-old woman weighing 130 and standing 5′ 5″ will maintain her weight by ingesting 2,070 calories per day, whereas her 45-year-old counterpart needs about 1,915.

One of the Internet resources enabling you to nail down daily calories needed for weight maintenance is the Diet Assessment Calorie Calculator in the website Calorie Control (www.caloriecontrol.org).

Diet Pills: NOT the Answer!

Athletes needing to lose pounds often ask if it's a good idea to take pills to facilitate or maintain weight loss. And each time I give them the same answer: Rarely is a pill the solution to a fitness problem. Most nutritional and fitness problems that arise can be thoroughly and affordably remedied through an effective Training Table program.

(The exception is when medicines are administered or recommended by a doctor.)

Reason One to Avoid Pills. Many over-the-counter diet pills have yet to undergo long-term objective clinical trials, and their efficacy in helping you to shed pounds largely remains unproven. Even the makers of adequately tested diet pills know what they are selling offers dubious results at best. If you don't believe it, look the fine print beneath the photo of the formerly obese middle-aged woman who now has a rock-solid body with six-pack abs. In almost every case you'll see the phrase "results not typical" – the manufacturer's safeguard against litigation by dissatisfied customers.

Reason Two. Diet pills don't work in the long term. Most studies show that any pill-induced weight loss is short lived – and once you stop taking the drug, you often pack on more pounds than you had before you began.

Reason Three. Diet pills can be very expensive, largely because the marketing blitzes that tout them are usually anything but cheap.

The Bottom Line: To maximize your overall fitness and athletic potential, you want solutions that last a lifetime, not the latest quick-fix pill or fad diet. Think like an athlete: To reach your ideal weight and maintain it, continue to eat strategically, exercise, and stick with the program.

All Hail the Mighty Pizza

If you added only tomato sauce to a pizza crust, your calories and macronutrients per slice would roughly amount to 125 calories, 25g carbs, 5g protein, and 2g total fat. But it's the toppings that make pizza one of our most popular foods, and they're so numerous and varied that they range from full-of-fat to fat-free.

Note: All nutrition facts in this chart, which run from the highest-calorie toppings to the lowest, are based on 1 ounce of meat, poultry, fish, vegetables, fruits, or sauces – and what you see may surprise you. Also keep in mind that some toppings are used more sparingly than others, which affects the comparisons found below. For instance, the low-cal onions (12 calories per ounce) on your pizza have less than a third of calories in garlic (42 per ounce), yet are more calorific because more onions are piled onto the pie.

Bacon 153 CALORIES • 0.5g carbs • 10.5g protein • 12g total fat

Pesto 138 CALORIES • 1.4g carbs • 2.6g protein • 14g total fat

Pepperoni 135 CALORIES • 1.2g carbs • 6g protein • 11.7g total fat

Hard cheeses* 112 CALORIES • 0.5g carbs • 9g protein • 8g total fat

Semi-hard cheeses* 100 CALORIES • 1g carbs • 7g protein • 7.5g total fat

Semi-soft cheeses* 98 CALORIES • 0.5g carbs • 7g protein • 7.5g total fat

Pork salami (pork/beef combo) 94 CALORIES • 1g carbs • 6g protein • 6g total fat

Ground pork 83 CALORIES • 0g carbs • 7g protein • 2g total fat

Ground lamb 82 CALORIES • 0g carbs • 7g protein • 6g total fat

Ground beef 78 CALORIES • 0g carbs • 7g protein • 5g total fat

Beef salami 75 CALORIES • 1g carbs • 4g protein • 6g total fat

Soft cheeses* 73 CALORIES • 0.5g carbs • 5g protein • 7g total fat

Black olives 66 CALORIES • 3.8g carbs • 0g protein • 5.7g total fat

Ground turkey 66 CALORIES • 0g carbs • 8g protein • 4g total fat

Kielbasa (turkey/beef combo) 63 CALORIES • 1g carbs • 4g protein • 5g total fat

Anchovies 60 CALORIES • 0g carbs • 8.2g protein • 2.7g total fat

Ground chicken 53 CALORIES • 0g carbs • 7g protein • 3g total fat

Turkey salami 47 CALORIES • 0g carbs • 5g protein • 3g total fat

Ham 46 CALORIES • 1.1g carbs • 4.6g protein • 2.4g total fat

Avocado 45 CALORIES • 1.5g carbs • 0.6g protein • 4.2g total fat

Garlic 42 CALORIES • 0.4g carbs • 1.8g protein • 0.1g total fat

Sweet Italian sausage 42 CALORIES • 1g carbs • 1g protein • 2g total fat

Green olives 41 CALORIES • 1.1g carbs • 0.6g protein • 4.3g total fat

Tuna (white, canned in oil) 36 CALORIES • 0.5g carbs • 7g protein • 1g total fat

Smoked turkey 26 CALORIES • 0g carbs • 6g protein • 0g total fat

Shrimp 33 CALORIES • 0.5 gcarbs • 6.5 protein • 0.5g total fat

Curd cheeses* 24 CALORIES • 1g carbs • 3g protein • 2.5g total fat

Shiitake mushroom 16 CALORIES • 40g carbs • 0g protein • 0g total fat

Pineapple 15 CALORIES • 4g carbs • 1.5g protein • 0.1g total fat

Onions 12 CALORIES • 3g carbs • 0g protein • 0g total fat

Broccoli 10 CALORIES • 2g carbs • 0.7g protein • 0.1g total fat

Roasted red pepper (1 oz, bottled) 9 CALORIES • 4g carbs • 0g protein • 0g total fat

Bell pepper 8 CALORIES • 2g carbs;0g protein • 0g total fat

Eggplant 8 CALORIES • 2g carbs • 0.3g protein • 0.1g total fat

Jalapeño pepper 8 CALORIES • 1.5g carbs • 0.3g protein • 0.3g total fat

Portobello mushroom 7 CALORIES • 1g carbs • 1g protein • 0g total fat

Spinach 7 CALORIES • 0g carbs • 0.8g protein • 0.1g total fat

Green chile 5 CALORIES • 0.10g carbs • 0g protein • 0g total fat

Tomato 5 CALORIES • 1g carbs • 0g protein • 0.1g total fat

Zucchini 5 CALORIES • 1g carbs • 0.3g protein • 0.1g total fat

Calories in cheese types are averaged from the "Cheese, Please" list in Chapter 6, Your Weight-Gain Training Table.

For Baby Boomers and Beyond ...

Fiber is a senior citizen's friend, and in more ways than one. Available only from plant-based foods and supplements, fiber improves your gastrointestinal system and overall health by keeping you regular, warding off hemorrhoids, and even reducing your risk of heart disease and colon cancer. Fiber swells when it reaches the stomach and leads to a feeling of fullness, which in turn can dull hunger.

How Much Do You Need? Getting enough fiber isn't quite as easy as you might think. Even if you eat five servings of fruits, vegetables, and whole-grain foods each day, you still might be short of the recommended daily allowance (RDA) for fiber. Your body needs at least 20 grams of fiber each day, and preferably 30 grams.

Staying Regular. If the fiber in your Training Table isn't keeping you regular, I recommend doubling your daily intake of whole-grain products, leafy green vegetables, nuts, legumes, and fruits. Wheat bran and oat bran are exceptionally good fiber sources. Beans, peas, lentils, lima beans, apples, almonds, dried figs, and prunes also have plenty of fiber. If you partake of these foods and a week later your bowel movements haven't increased, then it may be time to reach for over-the-counter fiber supplements – the most popular of which are based on psyllium, which comes from the plantain plant.

What About Gas? Yes, fiber produces gas in your intestinal tract, but you can lessen the problem if you increase your fiber intake gradually.

Nutritionists advise adults to start by consuming 10 to 15 grams per day – then, so the body will have time to adjust, to work their way up to 25 to 35 grams per day over the course of three or four weeks.

If You're the Parent of a Pre-Teen …

A hard truth of modern life is that too many manufacturers use advertising to undermine what is best for us and for our children when it comes to grocery shopping. And, obviously, It's harder for these messages to reach children who play outside, go to soccer practice, take tennis lessons, or engage in any other activities that pry them away from the TV set. My wife and I have always shown our daughter how to make healthy food choices, and now that she's older she understands that television commercials are designed to appeal to her senses on a variety of levels.

Burger and Fries = Happy Children? For the moment, perhaps. But in reality, happy children = parents doing a good job of overseeing their child's diet. It's tempting to dismiss wily TV commercials as harmless, but remember that advertising made it possible for a small hamburger stand to explode into an international chain boasting "billions and billions served."

Today that company is making some of its food offerings more healthful – but any way you look at it, fast foods are a key factor in America's obesity epidemic. French fries, milkshakes, hot dogs, hamburgers, tacos, fried chicken, and other foods high in fat and cholesterol are served in large portions when most people need only a fraction of the meat they eat daily. Too much fast food also leads to an increased risk of diabetes, heart disease, and other serious health problems. On the kid front, obesity can affect children's self esteem and mark them as targets for bullying.

Cool It! One way to keep children's consumption of fattening food to a minimum is to carry a small cooler in the car when the family goes out for a few hours. You'll sidestep the drive-thru by loading the cooler with fruit, lean cold-cut sandwiches, sweet baby carrots, bottled water, boxed 100% fruit juice, and the like. Keep it all cool by tossing in a frozen bottle of water.

Delicious Alternatives

When it comes to kids' favorite foods, it's amazing how much difference just switching to an equally tasty but less fattening alternative can make in a child's weight.

High-Calorie Favorites: Alternative Snacks/Drinks

High-Cal Favorite	Tasty Substitute
Potato Chips	Baked Chips
Ice Cream	Popsicles Made with Real Fruit
Soft Drinks	100% Fruit Juice
Milkshakes	Fruit Smoothies
Microwaved Buttered Popcorn	Air-Popped Popcorn with Flavored Salt

Chapter 6

Your Weight-Gain Training Table

Savvy Ways to Add Pounds

---

y far the most frequent question I hear competitive athletes ask is, "How can I put on weight and build muscle mass?" The first part of the answer is simple arithmetic: Consuming 500 calories more per day than you burn will, on average, enable you to gain 1 pound in one week. But gaining weight can be no picnic if you aren't eating strategically. Some athletes find it hard to eat enough just to fuel their practices and workouts, much less consume an extra 500 calories of the right kind day in, day out.

The Right Stuff

You can probably guess the follow-up question of how to put on weight and add muscle mass: "Which foods should I reach for to gain the extra calories?" My answer is always the same: The key is to eat more whole grains, fruits, and vegetables – the best sources of the carbohydrates that fuel your muscles and allow them to work harder and longer. Protein from meats, nuts, and dairy products is essential as well, but shouldn't be ingested to the point of doing more harm than good (see "A Common Misconception" in Chapter 7, Feeding the Athlete in You.)

Fast Food Allowed? I say no, unless you order one of the salads almost all fast food chains have wisely put on the menu. It's true that fast food staples are often sky-high in calories, which can help you gain weight. But these calories are largely empty, meaning they're disproportionately high in fat and provide very few nutrients. Take glazed doughnuts: The glaze is almost 100 percent sugar and the flour is refined, eliminating much of the grain's natural goodness. On top of that, doughnuts are fried, often in unhealthful saturated or trans fats.

"Weight" It Out. Weightlifting and other resistance exercises are also part of the weight-gain equation, causing the two types of skeletal muscle fibers in your body – fast-twitch and slow-twitch muscles – to grow in size and increase their glycogen-storage capacity. Here's the difference:

- **Fast-twitch muscles** are those you use for quick, powerful movements.
- **Slow-twitch muscles** control breathing and bodily activities during long distance running and other tests of endurance.

Whatever the type, bigger muscles understandably weigh more, thereby increasing your body weight in the way you want, not with more or larger fat cells.

Patience is key to increasing muscle mass. For most athletes who need to gain weight, adding about one-half to one pound a week is an attainable and responsible goal. Building up mass is much like running a marathon: Check how you're doing every so often to ensure that you're on pace, but not so frequently that it distracts you from the business at hand. (For more on exercise, see Chapter 10, Working Out, Weighing In.)

All things considered, enjoy your meals. Enjoy your snacks. Incorporate your favorite foods into your Training Table. But if you weigh yourself more than once a week, the readings on the scales may be useless. Why? Because it's only natural for weight to fluctuate as your body adjusts to a new eating plan, as discussed in Chapter 10.

--- *Take Note* ---

The Benefits of Building Muscle

Increased muscle size does more than just supply the power to hit a ball harder, wrestle your opponent to the mat, or beat your opponent to the basket. It also gives you stamina. More muscle mass means larger stores of glycogen, which serves as instant fuel for your muscles.

Think of your muscles as fuel tanks: The larger they are, the greater capacity they have to store ready-to-burn fuel. Building them up will help add mass to your frame and lead to better, longer-lasting performance no matter what your sport or physical activity. (See also "Best Time to Bulk Up" in Chapter 10, Working Out, Weighing In.)

--- • ---

Carbs to Choose, Fats to Shun

Do you need to eat constantly if you want to gain weight? Not quite, though it might seem so at times. And, while eating 35 times a week is central to your Training Table program, you may have to add a late-night snack each day, as shown in the Weight-Gain Training Table chart in Chapter 4.

To succeed, you obviously must take in more calories per day than you expend – in particular, *complex carbohydrates* from such foods as cereals, whole-wheat bread, and vegetables.

Simple carbohydrates include fructose (fruit sugar), sucrose (table sugar), lactose (milk sugar), and dietary fiber. Among the foods especially high in simple carbs are dates, raisins, dried apricots, and other dried fruits.

As mentioned above, for every 500 calories you consume above what you exert each day, you'll gain an average of a pound a week – and the wisest way to put on those 16 ounces is to up your portions of complex carbs with every meal and snack.

Best Complex Carb Sources. Foods high in complex carbs run the gamut. To make sure you're getting what you need, eat plenty of whole-wheat pastas, cereals, and breads. Cook up some green peas, sweet potatoes, and the corn-and-lima bean dish called succotash. Add an extra potato to your menu. Eat tortillas, rice, oatmeal, cream of wheat, and grits. (Note to northerners: Stir grated cheese into grits when they're almost done, and I promise that any preconceived notions about grits will evaporate with the first bite.)

Also make a point of venturing beyond your dietary comfort zone. Use different greens in your salads and then add beans, peas, celery, and carrots to the mix.

About Fat. Foods high in complex carbs are generally low fat – which brings up the place of fat in your diet. While some fat is essential, be particularly careful to avoid foods containing saturated fats and trans fats, which increase the risk or heart disease and stroke. In particular, banish foods fried in animal fat (lard or shortening). As for butter, use it sparingly, if at all.

Maintaining the Gain

It's important to view your Training Table as a dynamic tool that changes as your needs change. At the same time, once you've reached your target weight it's time to switch to maintenance mode.

Because humans are creatures of habit, eating patterns can prove to be stubborn to break. As I often remind the athletes I work with, gaining weight is a temporary endeavor, so they should enjoy it while they can. It's particularly hard to go from eating all we want while in the weight-gain mode to scaling back. But if we don't, surplus body fat will sabotage our athletic performance and even our health. For this reason, an effective weight-gain Training Table includes an extra step: summoning up your will power and self discipline!

Cheese, Please

The 40 cheeses in this chart run from highest in total fat to lowest – the reason the number of calories and the grams of carbohydrates and protein are rounded off but total fat is the more precise amount cited by the USDA National Nutrient Database. Note that soft cheeses like neufchâtel and soft goat cheese have less fat than hard and semi-soft types, and curd cheeses have the least. Note:

Calorie and macronutrient counts are based on 1 ounce of cheese.

Hard goat cheese 128 calories • 0.5g carbs • 9g protein • 10.19 TOTAL FAT

Kraft® 100% Parmesan Cheese 110 calories • 1g carbs • 4.75 protein • 9.50g TOTAL FAT

Cheddar 115 calories • 0.5g carbs • 7g protein • 9.40 TOTAL FAT

Gruyère 117 calories • 0g carbs • 8.5g protein • 9.17g TOTAL FAT

Colby 118 calories • 0.75g carbs • 6.5g protein • 9.10g TOTAL FAT

Fontina 110 calories • 0.5g carbs • 7.25g protein • 8.83g TOTAL FAT

Havarti 112 calories • 0.75g carbs • 6g protein • 8.80g TOTAL FAT

Roquefort 105 calories • 0.5g carbs • 6g protein • 8.69g TOTAL FAT

Monterey Jack 106 calories • 0.25g carbs • 7g protein • 8.58g TOTAL FAT

Semi-soft goat cheese 105 calories • 0.5g carbs • 7g protein • 8.52g TOTAL FAT

Muenster 105 calories • 0.25g carbs • 6.5g protein • 8.52g TOTAL FAT

Asiago 110 calories • 1g carbs • 8.5g protein • 8.44g TOTAL FAT

Brick 105 calories • 0.75g carbs • 6.5g protein • 8.41 TOTAL FAT

Caraway 107 calories • 1g carbs • 7g protein • 8.28g TOTAL FAT

Gorgonzola 100 calories • 2.5g carbs • 6g protein • 8.18 TOTAL FAT

Blue cheese (generic) 100 calories • 0.5g carbs • 6g protein • 8.15g TOTAL FAT

Parmesan 120 calories • 1g carbs • 11 protein • 8.11 TOTAL FAT

Edam 100 calories • 0.5g carbs • 7g protein • 7.88g TOTAL FAT

Swiss 108 calories • 00g carbs • 7.5g protein • 7.88g TOTAL FAT

Brie 95 calories • 1.5g carbs • 7g protein • 7.85g TOTAL FAT

Gouda 101 calories • 0.5g carbs • 7g protein • 7.78g TOTAL FAT

Romano 110 calories • 1g carbs • 9g protein • 7.64g TOTAL FAT

Jarlsberg 100 calories • 1g carbs • 7.5g protein • 7.60g TOTAL FAT

Provolone 100 calories • 0.5g carbs • 7.25g protein • 7.55g TOTAL FAT

Tilsit 96 calories • 0.5g carbs • 7g protein • 7.37g TOTAL FAT

Whole milk mozzarella 90 calories • 7.5g carbs • 6g protein • 6.99g TOTAL FAT

American (processed cheese) 93 calories • 2g carbs • 5.5g protein • 6.97g TOTAL FAT

Camembert 84 calories • 0g carbs • 5.5g protein • 6.88g TOTAL FAT

Neufchâtel 72 calories • 1g carbs • 2.5g protein • 6.46g TOTAL FAT

Feta 75 calories • 1.15g carbs • 4g protein • 6.03g TOTAL FAT

Soft goat cheese 75 calories • 0g carbs • 5g protein • 6g TOTAL FAT

Part skim mozzarella 72 calories • 0.75g carbs • 7g protein • 4.1 TOTAL FAT

Soy Kaas (soy cheese alternative) 60 calories • 1g carbs • 6g protein • 4.0g TOTAL FAT

Whole milk ricotta 50 calories • 1g carbs • 2g protein • 3.67g TOTAL FAT

Boursin 40 calories • 0.75g carbs • 3.5g protein • 2.50g TOTAL FAT

Part skim ricotta 40 calories • 1.5g carbs • 3g protein • 2.24g TOTAL FAT

Kraft® Velveeta (processed cheese) 40 calories • 1.5g carbs • 3g protein • 2.24g TOTAL FAT

4% milkfat cottage cheese 28 calories • 1g carbs • 3 g protein • 1.21 TOTAL FAT

2% milkfat cottage cheese 25 calories • 1g carbs • 3.5g protein • 0.69 TOTAL FAT

Nonfat cottage cheese 20 calories • 2g carbs • 3g protein • 0g TOTAL FAT

Feeding the Athlete in You

Making Each Bite Count

Diets are famous for promising quick results – and extreme promises usually call for extreme measures. Some diets frown on carbohydrates and tout high protein intake instead. Others call for mega-doses of vitamins or enzymes. A few even focus on a single fruit or vegetable (grapefruit, lychee, cabbage … you name it).

Whatever their claims, virtually all fad diets fall woefully short of providing you with the nutritional balance you need. The result is a two-headed hydra. Your body inevitably craves what it is has been denied (especially fat), so you fall off the wagon – and, in turn, compromise your workouts and athletic performance. The fact is, there's no middle ground: Food can be either an ally for the athlete in you or an obstacle sandbagging your progress.

Three things combine to bring your diet into balance: 1) The variety of foods you eat; 2) the number of calories you take in and how many you burn each day; and 3) the ratio of carbs, protein, and fat in your diet, which changes according to your short-term needs.

The Virtues of Variety

Many of the athletes I've advised once believed that loading up on vitamins and nutritional boosters like brewer's yeast, daily multivitamins, or whey protein powder meant they were not only taking good care of their bodies but also could eat whatever they craved – junk food included. They were mistaken. In fact, the trick is to eat a wide variety of foods.

How Do You Spell "Phytochemical"?

Varying your diet helps ensure you receive all the nutrients you need, including vitamins, minerals, trace elements, fiber, and phytochemicals. And what are phytochemicals? Simply put, plant chemicals containing protective, disease preventing

compounds. The countless phtytochemical catego-
ries and sub-categories are beyond the scope of this
book and, for almost everyone except biochemis-
try majors, a recipe for confusion. Mother Nature
offers a clue, however: Many phytochemicals are
pigments, imparting color that makes their food
sources relatively easy to identify.

For instance, the caretenoid we know as *beta-
carotene* is the compound that colors carrots, winter squash, and sweet potatoes orange; another
caretenoid, *lycopene*, makes tomatoes red. *Chlorophyll*
is responsible for the green of avocados, honeydew
melon, broccoli, string beans, zucchini, spinach,
lettuce, and other green fruits and vegetables. The
colors from *flavonoids* range across the spectrum,
and flavonoid-rich foods are usually full of healthful antioxidants. A good rule of thumb? The darker
the color of fruits and vegetables, the more antioxidants and vitamins they will supply.

Learning to Like New Foods

While lengthening your list of favorite foods
sounds like a simple task, without a concentrated effort it's all too easy to fall back on the old
standbys – and, in turn, deny yourself the better

nutrition that comes with variety. Still, I like what I see every year when it comes to changes in my athletes' food preferences. While as freshmen they arrive on campus relying on a fairly narrow range of foods, they leave with their culinary horizons greatly broadened.

Get Out of Your Rut. Much of our reluctance to try new foods has to do with what we ate growing up. Maybe your family had meat or poultry at every meal and gave short shrift to fruits and vegetables. Or perhaps you decided years ago that you simply didn't like broccoli, bananas, or beets. Old habits die hard, but one of the worst for a health-conscious person to keep is putting the same-old, same-old on the table day in and day out.

Look at it this way: It's almost certain that there's some part of your training program that you're not all that fond of, whether push-ups or abdominal crunches or the 40-minute walk you strike out on each day. But you get through it because you know what it does for your fitness and performance. Applying the same kind of discipline to expanding your menu is an important component of your Training Table. So don't be afraid to give new foods a try!

--- *Take Note* ---

You've Gotta Have Sole

Yes, you need to be eating sole — and also cod, haddock, catfish, and any other white flaky fish rich in low-fat protein and vitamin B 12. The same goes for firmer, oilier fish like salmon, trout, mackerel, and herring, which provide beneficial omega-3 fatty acids as well.

As healthful as fish is, I've found that many athletes just don't like it. This may include you, but you'll reap big rewards if you open your mind to the nutritional benefits of freshwater fish and seafood. While some are hardly low in fat (carp, for example, has 10 grams of fat per 6-ounce fillet, and Pacific herring has a whopping 22 grams per 6-ounce fillet), all are rich in cell-building proteins and other nutrients. Another plus: The fat in most fish is largely unsaturated, unlike fat in red meat and poultry.

To develop a taste for fish, start with filet of sole or another "non-fishy" type. Flavor it with seasonings you like, and then grill it. Or mix water-packed canned tuna into a healthy tomato-based pasta sauce. You'll barely know it's there!

--- • ---

The Skinny on Carbs, Protein, and Fat

With smart food choices in mind, let's take a closer look at carbohydrates, protein, and fat – the three macronutrients essential for growth and health.

Carbohydrates

Despite what the promoters of some diets lead you to believe, the bulk of your calories should come from carbs, especially if you're an active athlete. This is because carbohydrates (a blanket term for sugar, starch, and cellulose) are the organic compounds your body most easily converts into the energy fueling activity.

The Two Types of Carbs. Go for the simple, complex, or both?

Simple carbs (among them the sugars glucose and fructose) typically taste sweet and often have negligible value beyond calories. But does that mean you should always avoid them? When it comes to athletics, the answer is a qualified "No." Though they're the source so-called empty calories in table sugar, sodas, and candy, such calories are easy to digest and can be just what you need in the short term — when you play an intense tennis match, for example, or run a 5K footrace.

Complex carbs (starch, fiber) are abundant in whole-grain products and vegetables – particularly foods like potatoes and grains. These carbs provide the longer-lasting energy for endurance, but that's hardly their only virtue. Complex carbs also supply the vitamins and minerals essential to bodily processes, including B vitamins to build red blood cells and magnesium to aid bone growth.

Bottom Line on Carbs. Carbohydrates have been called the athlete's best friend. Simple carbs provide the burst of energy every athlete needs on occasion, and the complex carbs provided by grains, fruits, and vegetables can keep you going for the long haul.

Protein

Protein is composed of numerous amino acids and is used by your body much as a mason uses bricks and mortar. In fact, it's largely what we're made of. The same is true for animals as well, which is why beef, fish, pork, poultry, and dairy products are the best sources of this vital building block.

Consuming protein in all meals and snacks keeps the body in an anabolic (muscle-building) state. And eating snacks containing both protein and carbs is beneficial before and after strength-training workouts. As a bonus, protein intake can create a feeling of fullness, a plus when you're trying to keep your hunger and weight in check.

How Much Do You Need? It isn't hard to get enough protein: The daily requirement of calories-from-protein is 15 to 20 percent your caloric intake, and each gram of protein supplies 4 carbs. It's also easy to "do the math":

Calculations by the United States Department of Agriculture's show we need 0.36g of protein for every pound of body weight. Accordingly, if you weigh 150 pounds you'll want to consume around 55 grams of protein each day – an amount you would reach simply by having oatmeal for breakfast (about 7g), grilled vegetables and a cup of yogurt for lunch (16g), a handful of almonds in the afternoon (6g), and salmon with a side of broccoli for dinner (25g). Just don't overdo it, since a daily intake of 30 percent or more can do much more harm than good. (See "A Common Misconception" on the opposite page.)

Complete vs. Incomplete Protein. A protein source supplying all of the essential amino acids – animal-based foods like meat, poultry, fish, and dairy products – is called a *complete*, or high-quality, protein. Plant foods (fruits, vegetables, grains, nuts, and so on) provide *incomplete* protein, which lacks (or is low in) one or more of the essential amino acids.

Combine foods with complete and incomplete protein and you have complementary protein, which gives you all the amino acids you need. The reason rice and beans, both incomplete protein foods, have long been considered a perfect pairing is that in combo they supply the essential acids.

A Common Misconception. A passing knowledge of the fact that amino acids in protein build muscle mass and help repair injured body parts can lead to a widespread misconception – to wit, "the more protein, the better." Loading up on protein at the expense of carbs can put your metabolism into overdrive and cause ketosis – the body's burning of its own fat in place of the carbohydrates it ordinarily burns.

A daily calories-from-protein intake of 15 to 20 percent (1 gram protein = 4 calories) is enough to meet the needs of even the most demanding athlete. You enter the ketosis danger zone when your intake of protein averages out to 30 percent or more of daily caloric intake over time. The result is strain on your kidneys and heart, along with ketosis-based side effects such as dehydration, bad breath, and dizziness.

Bottom Line on Protein. Make sure you get enough complete or complementary protein by mixing and matching foods, but a daily calories-from-protein intake averaging 30 percent or more is something to avoid at all costs.

--- *Take Note* ---

Red Meat in a Woman's Diet

The female athletes I work with tend to favor skinless chicken, pork, tofu, and the like over the steaks and burgers. But I urge them to include at least a little red meat in their meals. Women need iron-rich foods to compensate for the blood lost during menstruation, and iron is abundant in red meats. (Other good iron sources include liver, clams, spinach, and beans.)

Still, a "moderation in all things" approach to red meat is wise. A Harvard School of Public Health study released in 2006 found that pre-menopausal women who ate red meat at least five times a week increased their risk of hormone receptive positive breast cancer, the most common form of the all-too-common disease. A good rule of thumb for women is to limit red meat to two meals a week, and choose lean cuts to reduce saturated fat intake.

--- • ---

Fat

As a food source, fat gets a bad rap, largely because of its high caloric content — 9 calories per gram, just over twice the calories from carbs and protein — and its association with high cholesterol. Yet it's an essential component of our diet. Besides giving flavor and substance to food, fat plays a vital role in the maintenance of cell membranes and furnishing the healthful fatty acids your body needs. It also keeps your skin from drying out and aids the body's absorption of vitamins A, D, E, and K. And, as my athletes soon realize, it supplies the substantial energy needed when playing sports, practicing, and exercising.

That said, it takes so little fat to meet your nutritional requirements that you needn't go out of your way to find it. Fat is abundantly present in dietary staples such as meat, dairy products, and vegetable oils. What's important to understand is the effects of good fats versus bad fats.

Good Fats. Unsaturated, or "good," fats come in three types:

Monounsaturated fats come from avocados, cashews, olives, peanuts, and certain other plant sources, yet much of the monounsaturated fat we consume is from olive oil and peanut oil used for cooking. On the health front, monounsaturated fats help reduce LDL, or "bad" cholesterol.

Polyunsaturated fats come from, among other plant sources, almonds, corn, cottonseeds, sesame seeds, safflower seeds, soybeans, sunflower seeds, and walnuts. Polyunsaturated fats reduce blood cholesterol because they promote the transport of HDL ("good" cholesterol) and discourage the formation of LDL.

Omega-3 fatty acids. Found in oily fish like salmon, tuna, mackerel, and sardines — and in lesser amounts in some plant sources (walnuts, flaxseed, and evening primrose oil among them) — omega-3 fatty acids have been shown to aid brain health. They also contribute to cardiovascular health by acting as an anti-inflammatory and anticoagulant.

Note: If you decide to add fish oil capsules to your daily regimen to increase your intake of omega-3, buy only from a reputable manufacturer that guarantees the fish oil capsules are 100 percent mercury-free.

Bad Fats. The kind to avoid, of which there are two:

Saturated fats. Unlike unsaturated fats, saturated fats prompt the liver to produce LDL, thereby increasing blood cholesterol levels. And, sad to say, the fat in many of our favorite foods – including meat, poultry, milk, butter, cheese, eggs, and most chocolate – is saturated. (A tip: It's easy to tell a saturated fat from an unsaturated fat because the former becomes solid at room temperature.)

Tropical oils – coconut oil, palm oil, and palm kernel oil – are sky-high in saturated fat. In fact, coconut oil has 40 percent more saturated fat than butter, reason enough to always check the ingredients to see if one of these oils is present.

Trans fats. While trans fats occur naturally in the milk of cows and sheep (though in very small quantities), partially hydrogenated versions account for almost all of the trans fats we consume. When it comes to fast food, French fries, and doughnuts are loaded with trans fats; in the supermarket, it's commonly used in baked goods to extend shelf life.

The elevated risk of coronary heart disease associated with trans fats has gained so much attention that product labels must now specify trans fat content, and a number of fast food chains no longer use hydrogenated cooking oils for frying. In addition, "No Trans Fats!" claims are often seen on food packaging nowadays. But guess what? By law, 0.5g or less of trans fat per serving equates with "none," so it's quite possible to ingest a few grams of trans fat each day without knowing it. The way to tell? If the list of ingredients on a label includes the words "partially hydrogenated," the food isn't entirely trans-fat free.

A Plus for Fat. With its many healthful benefits and potential pitfalls, fat also has another effect: It helps you to feel full longer because its molecular and nutritional complexity move it through your digestive tract more slowly than carbohydrates and protein. At the same time, fat can actually slow the absorption of carbs, so it's wise to avoid it when you're trying to replenish your glycogen stores immediately after exercise.

Bottom Line on Fat. To increase your intake of unsaturated fats and decrease saturated fats and trans fats, eat more grilled chicken (no skin), lean cuts of beef, broiled fish, avocados, olives, and nuts. Stay away from fried foods, and cut back on butter and creamy salad dressings.

The Importance of Vitamins and Minerals

No discussion of sports nutrition is complete without the role of vitamins and minerals, or *micronutrients*. To use an analogy, foods high in micronutrients are the equivalent of high-octane gas that burns cleanly and efficiently, whereas those low micronutrients are more like second-rate fuel.

Your Intricate Machine

The human body is a complicated machine made up of delicate systems that flourish only when they work in harmony. For that to happen, you need a regular supply of 13 vitamins and 16 minerals. In fact, without these non-caloric substances, your bodily systems would simply shut down. Your bones would become brittle, your central nervous system wouldn't send impulses to and from your brain, and sugars wouldn't be converted to glucose for energy. Moreover, your immune system wouldn't stave off infection and your blood wouldn't carry oxygen to your muscles, tissues, and organs.

Making it Tick. Hamburgers with fries will deliver protein, carbs, iron, and starch, (and a whole lot of saturated fat you don't want!), but they won't supply any calcium, copper, fluoride, or a bevy of other important minerals; nor will they give you many of the vitamins your body demands.

Even nutritious fruits, vegetables, and whole-grain products fall short of providing every micronutrient required for human life. It takes a variety of foods to incorporate all of these micronutrients into your daily diet and make your body tick. (See also "The Virtues of Variety," page 96.)

The 13 Essential Vitamins

Though your body manufacturers some vitamins, most must come from food – and any deficiency can result in serious disease. The list that follows notes each vitamin's function(s) and common food sources. Note: A few B vitamins are better known their common name (e.g., Niacin, Riboflavin) and are listed as such.

Biotin. Aids metabolic processing of carbohydrates; said to harden nails and aid hair growth. Sources: Egg yolks, soy products, fortified breakfast cereals

Folic acid (Folate, vitamin B9). Aids the production of red blood cells. Sources: Liver, egg yolks, spinach, kale, broccoli, avocados, legumes, fortified cereal products

Niacin (vitamin B3). Promotes growth and reduces cholesterol; helps the body's metabolization of carbs. Sources: Red meat, poultry, seafood, dairy products, eggs, legumes, whole grain products, fortified breakfast cereals

Pantothenic acid (vitamin B5). Maintains blood sugar levels; helps create antibodies, hemoglobin, and some hormones; helps the body's metabolization of carbs. Sources: Most foods, especially meats, whole grain products, avocados, broccoli

Riboflavin (vitamin B2). Helps kidney function; helps the body's metabolization of carbs. Sources: whole grain products, fortified breakfast cereals, red meat, poultry, dairy products, raw mushrooms

Thiamine (vitamin B1). Aids digestion, appetite, and nerve function; helps the body's metabolization of carbs. Sources: Pork, legumes, fortified breakfast cereals, whole grain products

Vitamin A. Helps keep skin, hair, and nails healthy; prevents night blindness. Sources: Liver, cold water fish (e.g., salmon, halibut, trout), fortified dairy products

Vitamin B6 (Pyridoxine). Aids metabolism, energy, nerve function, and growth of red blood cells. Sources: Red meat, fish, poultry, whole grain products, leafy green vegetables, potatoes, tofu and other soy products

Vitamin B12 (Cobalamin). Helps create red blood cells and nerve fibers. Sources: Red meat, fish, pork, poultry, seafood, dairy products

Vitamin C. Stimulates immune system; strengthens blood vessel walls; regulates cholesterol; promotes iron absorption. Sources: peppers, citrus fruits, guavas, melons, berries, broccoli

Vitamin D. Critical to the absorption of calcium and the health of teeth and bones. Sources: Fortified dairy products, cold-water fish (e.g., salmon, halibut, trout), sunlight

Vitamin E. Aids in maintaining muscle and building red blood cells; as an antioxidant, keeps cells healthy by warding off damaging oxidation. Sources: Eggs, vegetable oils, nuts, seeds, fortified breakfast cereals, leafy green vegetables

Vitamin K. Helps blood to clot. Sources: Leafy green vegetables, pork, green tea

The 16 Essential Minerals

Minerals (among them calcium copper, and magnesium) and trace elements (including iron, zinc, and selenium) are as important as vitamins, but they are required in minuscule amounts.

Calcium. Builds strong bones and teeth. Aids nerve function, blood clotting, and metabolism. Sources: Dairy products, tofu and other soy products, dark green vegetables

Chloride. Electrolyte essential for maintaining the body's proper acid-base balance and the production of digestive juices. Sources: Table salt, seafood, dairy products, red meat

Chromium. Works with insulin to metabolize glucose. Sources: Whole grain products, liver, brewer's yeast

Copper. Aids the absorption of iron; essential for maintenance of red blood cells, connective tissue, central nervous system, and skin pigment. Sources: Liver, shellfish, legumes, nuts, prunes

Fluoride. Aids bone and tooth strength. Sources: Tea, fluoridated water

Iodine. Essential for formation of thyroid hormones and regulation of metabolism. Sources: Iodized table salt, seafood, seaweed

Iron. Helps transport oxygen through the body. Sources: Liver, red meat, seafood, legumes, fortified breakfast cereal

Manganese. Critical to the repair of tendons and bones; aids metabolism. Sources: coffee, tea, legumes

Magnesium. Aids in bone growth and helps muscles function efficiently. Sources: Leafy green vegetables, legumes, whole grain products, red meat, poultry, fish, eggs

Molybdenum. Aids metabolism and storage of iron. Sources: Organ meats, leafy green vegetables (dark), whole grain products

Phosphorus. Helps bones and teeth stay strong; aids metabolism. Sources: Red meat, poultry, fish, eggs, legumes, dairy products

Potassium. Electrolyte aiding the maintenance of fluid balance, muscle function, and metabolism. Sources: Avocados, bananas, citrus fruits, legumes, whole grain products

Selenium. As an antioxidant, keeps cells healthy by warding off damaging oxidation. Sources: Poultry, seafood, organ meats, whole grain products, legumes

Sodium. Electrolyte aiding the maintenance of fluid balance and muscle function. Sources: Table salt, dairy products, seafood, processed foods

Sulfur. Component of B vitamins and several amino acids; found in every cell but is concentrated in skin, hair, and nails. Sources: Red meat, poultry, pork, fish, legumes, nuts

Zinc. Helps enzymes to function; aids in cellular reproduction and growth. Sources: Oysters, red meat, yogurt, tofu, fortified breakfast cereals

What About Supplements?

Are vitamin and mineral supplements necessary to ensure that you receive each micronutrient in proper quantities? Probably not. While I don't have a hard-nosed position against multivitamins, they aren't typically required for anyone whose Training Table incudes foods from across the spectrum.

Exceptions to the Rule

Nevertheless, there will be times when there's good cause to take a supplement – one being ferrous sulfate (iron) to treat anemia. In addition, there's no harm in taking multivitamins once a day. Just remember that they don't offer carbs, fat, or protein, and they certainly won't provide any fiber. Also bear in mind that a variety of colorful and nutritious food – not a handful of pills and capsules – is the foundation of an effective Training Table.

For Baby Boomers and Beyond ...

Luckily, modern science is discovering which trace elements, antioxidants, and assorted other nutrients will benefit us all the more as we grow older.

Here, in alphabetical order, are four that anyone over 50 should pay attention to — and why.

Anthocyanin. This plant pigment gives dark red and dark blue foods their color. It also happens to be an especially powerful antioxidant. Studies have shown that anthocyanin helps guard against degenerative brain diseases, cardiovascular disease, and mood disorders. Among the best sources are red cabbage, beets, blueberries, blackberries, black currants, red or black grapes, pomegranates, and cranberries — and 100-percent juices are a good way to enjoy the benefits of these red or blue-black fruits (think hard-to-eat pomegranates).

Folic acid (vitamin B9). Folic acid, also known as folate, aids the proper function of the central nervous system and the production of red and white blood cells. It is also believed to slow the effects of aging on the brain. In addition, tests have shown it can lower high homocysteine levels in the blood, decreasing the risk of stroke and heart attack (homocysteine is an amino acid). Rich sources of folic acid include spinach, avocados, lentils and other legumes, foliate-fortified cereals, and liver.

Lutein. Lutein, a carotenoid antioxidant naturally present in the body, is highly concentrated in the macular region of the retina — so it's hardly surprising that it's been shown to protect against such age-related eye conditions as macular degeneration and cataracts. Tests have also shown lutein to increase skin hydration and elasticity and to aid the thickening of arterial walls. The best sources? Spinach, kale (along with other cabbage family members like broccoli and Brussels sprouts), romaine lettuce, leeks, and peas. By far the best animal source is the egg yolk, which provides lutein in a lipid form more easily absorbed by the body.

Omega-3. See "Good Fats," page 106.

If You're the Parent of a Pre-Teen ...

It should come as no surprise that parents who eat plenty of fruits and vegetables and have fried foods only as a rare indulgence are likely to raise kids who will do the same in their adult lives. Such a diet will also give youngsters the nutrients they need to fuel their active lifestyles and grow healthy muscles, strong bones, sharp minds, and hardy immune systems.

Speak up. Because teachers, babysitters, and the staff at day-care facilities might very well spend as much time with your child as you do, don't be afraid to bring up your child's preference for healthy meals and snacks. Tell them that you view cakes, cookies, and candy as an occasional indulgence (no more than one small treat per day, please); that carbonated beverages are off-limits (water, milk, and fruit juices only, thanks); and that fresh fruits, vegetables, and nutrition-packed peanut butter and jelly sandwiches are the preferred food choices. If necessary (or allowed), pack a lunch with the foods that will give your child the range of nutrients he or she needs.

Chapter 8

Building Endurance

Keeping Your Stamina Going

Endurance athletes don't just enjoy pushing their bodies and mental toughness to the limit: They thrive on it. I've helped many of them make the necessary adjustments to their Training Tables as they move from a lifetime of playing organized sports to training for a 42K (26.2-mile) marathon or other endurance sport.

Of course, you don't have to be a retired athlete or a marathon runner to enjoy the endurance-building aspect of a Training Table program. It applies equally to the young mother who's about to compete in an amateur tennis tournament, the 65-year-old who wants to go the distance in a touch football game with his grandkids, and the golfer who wants to make sure her energy doesn't flag when she plays two 18-hole rounds in one day.

Put Yourself in Steve's Shoes

To illustrate what it takes to build endurance before an athletic event, we'll focus on Steve, a former college athlete who consulted me when he was about to run his first marathon.

"Magic," Steve said, "I'm following a training schedule designed to help my performance peak on marathon day, but I seem to run out of gas during my longer runs."

Steve's complaint is something I've heard often, especially from former athletes who've been out of the gym for a few years and now have a new career and a family.

"Have you lost weight since your training began?" I asked him.

"Yes, but don't all marathoners? Who wants to lug 10 pounds of belly fat up and down hills for 42K?" It was true that Steve was already lean.

Along with losing weight, Steve was doing several other things right to prepare for his first marathon: He adhered to a diligent training schedule, wore the right shoes, ate balanced meals, and had ramped up his daily percentage of carbohydrates by making sure he had whole-wheat pasta once a day. But even these smart choices weren't enough. It was clear that Steve needed more calories to build endurance.

Steve Changes Course. It's no wonder that Steve described his long runs as grueling – he really was running out of gas. And this was hardly a surprise. Most of the time, endurance athletes don't go about ingesting carbs in the most effective way: During their training period and on race day, countless runners and bikers load up on huge bowls of pasta when there's no real need to gorge.

When I told Steve as much, he said, "That's good to hear," he said "So how should I eat?"

We spent the next few minutes talking about ways he could increase the fuel in his diet gradually and throughout the day. Add a pasta salad to lunch, for example. Have a peanut butter and jelly sandwich before a workout. Eat a banana after dinner. All of these carb-rich foods eliminate the need to "load up" on carbs in a mere one or two meals on the big day.

Steve phoned me a few weeks later, excited about how enjoyable his training had become – all because he no longer ran out of gas during long runs. Now that his training was back on track, I encouraged him to rebalance his intake of carbs, fat, and protein as he trained. He would gradually increase the proportion of carbs from around 65 percent of calories from carbs (rather than fat or protein) to around 75 percent on race day. This macronutrient rebalancing is the foundation of building endurance as well.

Take It Easier

It wasn't too long ago when well respected sports nutritionists advised marathon runners and other endurance athletes to completely drain the glycogen stores in their muscles and liver a week or so before the race or tournament. The athletes did so by depriving their bodies of most carbohydrates (simple and complex alike) and training hard to deplete their carbohydrate stores, or glycogen. They could then restock them through mega-doses as race day approached. The thinking was that your glycogen-deprived muscles would gorge on the sudden influx of glucose and store more fuel than usual.

It was an interesting idea and it worked. But research has shown that it's not the best approach, which is the reason I don't advise it. Your body neither likes, nor responds well to, abrupt changes in its physiology. Because the human body was molded by eons of the feast-or-famine life of the hunter-gatherers, it panics when its fuel is drained. With this in mind, your better course is to ramp up the percentage of calories-from-carbs in your Training Table with a diet consisting largely of pasta, vegetables, fruit, and whole grains.

Stick to the Usual

The same gradual approach applies to race or game day. Don't suddenly throw your body a curve by introducing new foods to the mix. For instance, If you've never eaten muesli, then don't start now! Maybe it has more fiber than your system is used to, causing cramping, gas, and not-so-pleasant stops in the roadside Port-a-John. Maybe it has more sodium, and drains your body of precious liquid. Instead, eat a breakfast of carbohydrate-rich foods you know you like, and in portions you know your system can tolerate.

--- *Take Note* ---

Pre-Race Food Testing

When preparing for a long race, it's a good idea to use your training days to test the timing and type of meal you'll have on the day of the run – a way to see what feels best to you. Have just enough food on your stomach to stay comfortable while keeping hunger pangs at bay. Then, on race day, eat what you know works best for you.

--- • ---

When (and What) to Drink

Now back to Steve. In addition to advising him to adjust his intake of carbs, fat, and protein, I encouraged him to prehydrate his body beginning 24 hours before the race – something vital to both health and performance. This involved filling two 2-liter bottles with water and drinking little by little over the course of the day before the race. Combined with the liquid Steve ingests through food, the water adequately hydrated his cells before the start of the race. (See "Drinks from Garden, Bush, and Tree" in Chapter 9, Hydration, Hydration, Hydration.). I also encouraged him to wash down his game day carb-heavy breakfast with water or, if he preferred, a sports drink.

Don't Wait for Thirst

My last bit of advice to Steve was the most important: not to wait until he felt thirsty before knocking back a few mouthfuls of fluid – and to do it repeatedly. I told him that "Drink before I get thirsty" should be his mantra.

It should be your mantra, too, when you participate in an endurance event. A good rule of thumb is to drink 5 ounces of fluid every 10 to 15 minutes, if possible. This will help to keep your body hydrated and cool your body temperature – and, if you're choosing a sports drink over water, it will help replenish the rapidly depleting glycogen stores in your muscles and liver. Replenishing blood glucose is critical to success, since most of us can store enough glycogen (your primary muscle fueler) for no longer than 90 minutes.

Hot Days = Health Risks

Remember that the hotter the air temperature, the quicker the fluids you drink are lost through sweat, waste removal, and breathing. Insufficient intake on a hot day puts you at risk of heat fatigue, heat stroke, and dehydration. Should any of these conditions affect you, heat becomes less about your performance and more a matter of serious health consequences – and even of survival.

Refueling During Activity

If your athletic activity lasts longer than 60–90 minutes, you need more than just bottled water. Sports drinks and the occasional snack – say, a banana or a few orange slices – will help keep your energy at the level you need.

Sports Drinks vs. Energy Drinks. How do sports drinks differ from energy drinks? Sports drinks are superior for endurance sports because they contain the right amount of electrolytes and carbohydrates, while energy drinks often merely provide jolts of caffeine and sugar. (For a comparison of water, sports drinks, and energy drinks, see "Water, or an Alternative?" in Chapter 9, Hydration, Hydration, Hydration.).

Chugging Down Carbs

Like everyone who lives in the South, Vanderbilt athletes drink a lot of iced tea, which is carb-free unless sweetened with sugar. Other beverages not only have carbs but fat – and not just in dairy products. The calories and macronutrients in common beverages are compared in this chart, with the list running from highest carb content to lowest; drinks with identical carb contents run alphabetically.

As a matter of interest, the list includes beverages that have little or no place in the athletic realm and, in fact, no macronutrients to speak of – coffee, tea, beer, wine, and what I and many other sports nutritionists consider the athlete's bane: soft drinks.

Note: Calorie and macronutrient amounts are based on an 8-ounce serving.

> **Red grape juice** 170 calories • 44g CARBS • 0g protein • 0g total fat
>
> **White grape juice** 160 calories • 39g CARBS • 0g protein • 0g total fat
>
> **Apricot nectar** 141 calories • 36g CARBS • 0.9g protein • .0.2g total fat

Pomegranate juice 145 calories • 36g CARBS • 0g protein • 0g total fat

Peach nectar 135 calories • 35g CARBS • 0.7g protein • 0g total fat

Pineapple juice 135 calories • 35g CARBS • 1g protein • 0.20g total fat

Mango juice 125 calories • 31g CARBS • 0 protein • 0g total fat

Cranberry juice 120 calories • 30g CARBS • 1g protein • 1g total fat

Fruit punch 1 20 calories • 30g CARBS • 0g protein • 0g total fat

Guava juice 120 calories • 29g CARBS • 0g protein • 0g total fat

Apple juice 116 calories • 28g CARBS • 1g protein • 0.3g total fat

Lemonade 105 calories • 28g CARBS • 0.15g protein • 0.2g total fat

Red Bull® 108 calories • 28g CARBS • 0g protein • 0g total fat

Coca-Cola Classic® 100 calories • 27g CARBS • 0g protein • 0g total fat

Root Beer 100 calories • 26g CARBS • 0g protein • 0g total fat

Orange juice 110 calories • 25g CARBS • 1.25g protein • 0.15g total fat

Rice milk 125 calories • 25g CARBS • 00g protein • 00g total fat

Chocolate milk (whole) 172 calories • 25g CARBS • 8g protein • 8.5g total fat

Grapefruit juice 95 calories • 22g CARBS • 1.25g protein • 0.2g total fat

Cow's milk (whole) 145 calories • 13g CARBS • 8g protein • 8g total fat

Buttermilk (whole) 1 50 calories • 13g CARBS • 8.5g protein • 8g total fat

Cow's milk (2%) 120 calories • 12.5g CARBS • 8g protein • 5g total fat

Cow's milk (1%) 105 calories • 12.5g CARBS • 8.5g protein • 2.5g total fat

Cow's milk (nonfat/skim) 90 calories • 12.5g CARBS • 8.5g protein • 0.7g total fat

Goat's milk 140 calories • 11g CARBS • 8g protein • 7g total fat

Soy milk (plain) 115 calories • 10g CARBS • 7g protein • 4g total fat

Tomato juice 40 calories • 10g CARBS • 2g protein • 0.2g total fat

V8 Juice® 50 calories • 10g CARBS • 2g protein • 0g total fat

Coconut water 45 calories • 9g CARBS • 1.5g protein • 0.5g total fat

Beer (regular) 1 00 calories • 8.5g CARBS
1g protein • 0g total fat

Almond milk 60 calories • 8g CARBS • 1g protein • 2.5g total fat

Red table wine 190 calories • 6g CARBS • 1g protein • 0g total fat

Beer (light) 68 calories • 4g CARBS • 0.5g protein • 0g total fat

White table wine 130 calories • 4g CARBS • 1g protein • 1g total fat

Black tea 2 calories • 1g CARBS • 0g protein • 0g total fat

Chamomile tea 2 calories • 0.5g CARBS • 0g protein • 0g total fat

Herbal tea other than chamomile 2 calories • 0g CARBS • 0g protein • 0g total fat

Diet Coke® 1 calorie • 0.5g CARBS • 0g protein • 0g total fat

Coffee (black)*
Diet Pepsi®*
Green tea*

Contains neither calories nor macronutrients

Staving Off Heat Stress

Heat stress, usually brought on by a mix of high temperatures and exercise, is a condition marked by the onset of headache, dizziness, fatigue, a weak cough, or more shortness of breath than is usual. Whenever you suspect heat stress, don't wait for symptoms to escalate before taking these countermeasures:

- Go as quickly as possible to an air-conditioned or shady place.
- Sit or lie down.
- Drink several mouthfuls of cool water or sports drink.
- Shed heat-trapping polyester clothing.
- Apply cool, wet cloths to the head and neck area.

If the symptoms of heat stress fail to quickly subside, seek emergency medical attention immediately.

Chapter 9

Hydration, Hydration, Hydration

What – and When – to Drink

Naturally, one of the keys to a successful Training Table is taking in enough fluid. I encourage my athletes to carry a water bottle everywhere they go, not just on the field. It's that important. But guess what? Those 8 glasses of water we've long been told are essential to drink each day don't always come only from the faucet or supermarket. Many solid foods contain water (especially fruits and vegetables, as shown on the next two pages in "Drinks from Garden, Bush, and Tree"), and your daily intake of these watery foods – plus liquids like skim milk, juice, soup, and non-caffeinated beverages – help you to reach the daily requirement. Who knew that a roasted chicken breast is 65 percent water, and the water content of eggs is 75 percent?

Here are some other water-in-food percentages, most of which may surprise you:

- Popsicles and Jell-O®: 90 percent water
- Oysters: about 85 percent water
- Most other shellfish and fin fish such as salmon, trout, cod, haddock, and sole: about 75 percent water
- Most meats cooked rare to medium: 50 to 70 percent water
- Most meats cooked well done: 40 to 50 percent water
- Soft cheeses: about 60 percent water
- Hard cheeses, 35 to 50 percent water
- Most breads: about 35 percent water
- Most cakes: about 20 to 35 percent water

--- *Take Note* ---

Drinks from Garden, Bush, and Tree

Much of the water we need comes from fruits and vegetables. These water-content percentages (all but one from the University of Kentucky Cooperative Extension Service) are based on raw produce – but even when cooked these foods increase your daily fluid intake.

15 "Juiciest" Fruits

Lemon*: 96% water

Banana, strawberry, watermelon 92%

Grapefruit, lime, papaya: 91%

Cantaloupe: 90%

Passion fruit, peach, tangerine: 88%

Pineapple, raspberry: 87%

Apricot: 86%

Plum: 85%

*Source: Bowes and Church's Food Values of Portions Commonly Used

15 "Juiciest" Vegetables

Cucumber, iceberg lettuce: 96% water

Celery, radish, zucchini: 95%

Ripe tomato**: 94%

Green cabbage, green tomato: 93%

Bell pepper, cauliflower, eggplant, red cabbage, spinach: 92%

Broccoli: 91%

Carrot: 87%

**Botanically a fruit but eaten as a vegetable

___ • ___

Just How Much Fluid?

According to the National Research Council, a healthy adult needs around a fifth of a teaspoon of liquid for every calorie burned. As such, an athletic person who burns 2,900 calories needs to drink around 100 ounces of water each day, or about 12 1/2 cups. That's a lot, and it doesn't account for the water you lose from sweat when you exercise or whenever you're outside for extended periods of time during hot weather.

The truth is, most of us don't get enough of the wet stuff simply because we wait until we're thirsty before we reach for it – but by then, we're already in a performance-crunching catch-up mode. People in general, and athletes in particular, need to condition themselves to ingest fluids out of habit, not thirst, if they're going take in the copious amounts the human body needs.

And Why? Getting enough fluid, whether directly or indirectly, isn't a matter of choice. Water in any form is essential because it …

- Transports nutrients throughout the body and collects and removes waste
- Helps regulate body temperature through sweat

- Aids the absorption of nutrients
- Lubricates the joints
- Forms the basis for the plasma in blood
- Possibly reduces the risk for some forms of cancer

Sweat It!

In many ways, your body is like a high-performance car: Both require the right fuel to function at their peak, and they need to be constantly cooled to prevent overheating. When your muscles work, whether when you walk across the room or lift weights, heat is generated as a natural byproduct. So, to keep your body temperature cooler, you sweat. Without sweating, you couldn't survive.

Your Inner Cooler. How does sweating keep your body cool? By removing much of the excess heat from your body (something that waste removal and even breathing do as well). Even during periods of rest your body is busy cooling itself. Believe it or not, a healthy person is almost always sweating – though in lesser quantities than during times of physical exertion.

The Danger of Water Loss. As amazing as it seems, your body can produce up to three quarts of sweat per hour when you exert yourself in extreme conditions. That's why even in normal conditions it's critical to your performance (and, more important, your health) that you quickly replace the fluid lost to sweat and other bodily processes. If you don't, you risk suffering dehydration, circulatory problems, kidney failure, and heat stroke – or, as news reports during extreme heat waves show all too frequently, death.

The Two Types of Sweat

Did you know that your body actually produces two types of sweat? The average person has more than 2.5 million sweat glands in the skin, covering virtually the entire body. And the more active you are, the busier those sweat glands.

- **Eccrine Sweat.** Most sweat glands are of the eccrine type and produce sweat largely composed of water, sodium chloride, and a bit of potassium. Eccrine glands are particularly numerous on the forehead, the palm, and the soles of your feet.

- **Apocrine Sweat.** Sweat from the apocrine sweat glands, mostly found in the armpits and the anal/genital area, contains protein and fatty acids in addition to water, sodium chloride, and potassium – "extras" that give apocrine sweat a more viscous texture and a yellowish cast. This accounts for the yellow stains on the underarm areas of clothing.

––– *Take Note* –––

Signs of Dehydration

Because the earliest stages of dehydration are often difficult to detect, always drink before onset of thirst. Oddly, thirst isn't the first symptom to crop up as dehydration begins. Oftentimes the first signs are as varied as dry mouth, sticky saliva, flushed face, dry skin, disorientation, headaches, and weakness. Once any these occurs your ability to perform athletically is already compromised, so be sure to drink up daily.

––– • –––

The Importance of Prehydrating

As you lose fluids through sweat and waste removal, your body becomes stressed. In turn, your blood plasma thickens and makes it harder for your heart to pump blood and deliver nutrients throughout your body, remove waste, and help keep you cool. Not surprisingly, you become dehydrated.

Practice/Game Day Hydration. Here's the prehydrating process my athletes follow before (and during) practice sessions and on game day:

1) Five hours before the practice or game, they drink 20 ounces of water or sports drink to get the ball rolling (so to speak) – a few ounces less if they're on the skinny side, and about 30 ounces if they weigh in the mid-200s or more.

2) Two hours later, they drink the equivalent amount of fluid.

3) Fifteen minutes before the practice or game, the athletes drink five ounces of water or sports drink.

4) I also urge athletes to drink five ounces of fluid every 10 to 20 minutes once the practice or game is in progress, regardless of whether they feel thirsty.

Ingesting all this fluid enables the body to absorb and distribute it to the muscles, tissues, organs, and blood stream in advance – and taking it in gradually ensures an athlete's stomach won't have too much liquid sloshing around.

Do It Yourself. You can tailor this pre-hydration process to your own needs whenever you plan a bout of strenuous exertion. If, say, you've pre-hydrated yourself and stay thirsty even when drinking 5 ounces at regular intervals, increase your fluid intake to 8 ounces every 10 to 20 minutes. If you still feel dehydrated, drink 10 ounces of fluid every 15 minutes.

--- *Take Note* ---

Play, Weigh, Hydrate

Here's a way to make sure you replace fluid lost to sweat during practice, training, or playing a team sport or a one-one-one match: Weigh yourself both before the event and immediately afterwards. Then drink three cups of water or sports drink for every pound lost. It's that easy!

--- • ---

Water, or an Alternative?

Generally, water gives your body much of what it needs. But during times of exertion, the carbs and other substances in sports drinks do a terrific job helping to sustain your body's ability to perform at its best. So-called energy drinks, on the other hand, can be an iffy proposition.

Sports Drinks

Research has shown that a carbohydrate solution is ideal for hydrating the body and fighting fatigue during extended periods of exercise. And the manufacturers of Gatorade® and other sports drinks know how to maximize the impact: They calibrate the solution to provide six to eight grams per serving. Why so? Because ingesting any more will make it hard for your body to digest the carbs, whereas ingesting fewer grams won't give you what you need to get through the event.

Electrolytes Keep You Charged. Sports drinks do more than just deliver fatigue-fighting carbs and cool you off. They replace electrolytes (salts whose primary ions include sodium, potassium, magnesium, and other minerals), which we sweat out in great quantities as we exercise or compete in a game. These salts not only help the blood carry electrical impulses to your nerves and muscles but also help you absorb fluid quickly and retain it longer. Fortunately, the amount of salts in sports drinks is small enough to keep your tissues from swelling the way they do after you've eaten a salty meal.

Note: Make-your-own sports drinks are marketed in the form of electrolyte mixes or gels – so if you want to determine the salts content of your drink, just add water and shake or stir.

When to Drink. If you anticipate your exertion to last 90 minutes or longer, drink a sports beverage in steady, small amounts to help keep your blood glucose levels high and preserve muscle glycogen. Doing so has two big benefits: 1) you'll stave off dehydration by keeping your liquid reserves at safe levels, and 2) ingesting fluid in small amounts keeps you from weighing yourself down. (Can you imagine how you would feel if you were trying to do jumping jacks immediately after chugging 20 ounces of liquid?) When it comes to hydrating the body, the old axiom proves accurate: Slow and steady wins the race.

Energy Drinks

High-carb, high-calorie, high-caffeine beverages marketed as energy drinks can have a downside. While they make you more energetic in the short term, they could actually end up hampering your performance, depending on the ingredients they contain.

Caffeine's Bad Buzz. Whether it comes from coffee beans or the tropical plants guarana and kola nut (both with three times more caffeine than coffee), caffeine in energy drinks pulls much-needed moisture from your tissues. In many people, caffeine also causes undesirable gastrointestinal side effects – diarrhea, for one. Other side effects may include nervousness, insomnia, heart palpitations, and headache.

Many energy drinks are supplemented carbohydrates, vitamins, and minerals, so not all of them are to be avoided. The trick is to check the product label to be sure you'll get more than just a bone-rattling jolt of caffeine.

--- *Take Note* ---

Checking Your Water Level

I tell my athletes they can gauge whether they're getting enough water by paying close attention to their urine.

- *A pale-yellow or clear color generally indicates proper hydration.*
- *A dark-yellow color generally means more fluids are needed.*

The frequency of urination is also an indicator. If you urinate fewer than four times each day, you definitely need more fluid. When this is the case, up your intake by adding at least one extra cup of water, juice, or sports drink to each of your meals and snacks.

___ • ___

Hot vs. Cold

Which is better for an athlete to drink while competing or working out: room-temperature, cold, or warm liquid? Opinions vary, but it all boils down to common sense.

Cold and Iced Liquids. These bring down your body temperature, thus aiding your performance. At the same time, cold beverages can be hard to swallow in large quantities. Quickly downing iced liquids fast can also result in the short-lived but intense headache known as "brain-freeze." (FYI, brain-freeze is a response of the hypothalamus, a part of the brain that regulates body temperature.) Of course, brain-freeze is unlikely to occur if you adhere to my strategy of drinking 5 ounces of liquid every 10 to 20 minutes, therefore eliminating the need to chug-a-lug like there's no tomorrow.

Warm liquids. Nor surprisingly, these are preferable when you exercise or play sports outside on a very cold day and your body temperature may drop too low for your own good. When this is the case, I recommend drinking either room-temperature or warm water or some decaffeinated hot tea or hot chocolate.

Post-Game Fill-up. After the game, infuse your body with a lot more fluid, regardless of its temperature. For each pound of body weight lost during exertion, you need to drink 16 ounces of fluid.

For Baby Boomers and Beyond …

Besides the slowing of metabolism, other bodily changes occur as we age. For one, our ability to taste food and feel thirst decreases because our thirst-triggering mechanisms don't work as well.

Why bring up taste in a chapter devoted to hydration? Because taste and thirst are inextricably intertwined. When food tastes bland, we tend to add salt to bring out the flavors we've come to enjoy. Mashed potatoes don't have much flavor? Add salt. Soup a little bland? Add salt. The problem is, salt is a diuretic, meaning it pulls moisture out of your tissues and makes you thirsty.

Outpace Thirst. Thirst is normally a warning that dehydration is beginning to set in – but as we age, the warning bell doesn't ring until dehydration is advanced. This means that seniors often don't quench their thirst until their mouths are dry and the heart working harder to compensate for too little fluid. As a result, it's to your advantage to drink 8 ounces of non-caffeinated liquid every 90 minutes you're awake. If it's a particularly hot day, drink even more.

You'll want to steer clear of most soft drinks because caffeine – like salt – is a diuretic. Prefer milk? No problem, since it has a high water content. Fruit juices? Go for it. Sports drinks? Terrific. And, as "Drinks from Garden, Bush, and Trees" on page 136–137 shows, the water you get from many foods can go a long way toward topping you up.

If You're the Parent of a Pre-Teen …

It goes without saying that children are as much in need of pre-hydrating as adults. Follow this advice on the days your youngster sets off to play soccer, softball, or any other team sport: You and the coaches of your child's team should ensure that the youngsters drink small amounts of water or sports drink regularly throughout the game. Three or four large sips every 10 to 15 minutes is usually enough to keep dehydration at bay.

Chapter 10

Working Out, Weighing In
FREE Advice for Bulking Up

A s I've stressed in previous chapters, a Training Table program is about more than what you eat: The first "E" in FREE stands for "exercise." As an athlete, you may think your active lifestyle is exercise enough – but think again. No matter how strenuous a game, match, or round may be, sports alone won't do the trick.

Three or more times a week, you need to set aside a minimum of 30 minutes for some aerobic or resistance exercise, whether jogging, walking, cycling, doing sit ups and push ups, or working out at the gym. Aerobic exercise is essential, but I also recommend two weekly sessions of muscle-strengthening resistance exercise.

Regular exercise improves your life in almost too many ways to count. The major benefits include making the heart and lungs work more efficiently, lowering cholesterol and blood pressure, reducing the risk of diabetes, increasing mental acuity, and giving you more energy. You'll also get a better night's sleep and gain an overall sense of well-being.

Aerobic vs. Resistance Exercise

Aerobic exercise, which includes jogging, brisk walking, cycling, and skiing, calls on large muscle groups to function and causes the heart and lungs to work much harder than they do during periods of inactivity – hence its other name: cardiovascular exercise. Whatever you call it, it's an excellent way of strengthening your heart and keeping your circulatory system, which delivers oxygen throughout the body, in good working order.

Just be sure you have enough carbohydrates in your system when doing aerobic exercise, since carbs create the glycogen and blood sugar responsible for fueling muscles. It may surprise you to learn that when your system is low in carbs, exertion that would otherwise benefit the body can actually be counterproductive. How so? Because when your body is deprived of carbs, muscles sometimes begin to convert their protein into the energy your body cries out for.

Resistance exercise includes weightlifting, push-ups, squats, and some forms of yoga and Pilates. Resistance builds muscle strength and mass by overworking specific muscles and strengthening them gradually over a period of weeks and months. While this kind of exercise adds weight to your frame by adding muscle instead of fat, resistance exercises are less effective than aerobic exercise when it comes to cardiovascular and pulmonary health.

Calories and Exercise

When starting a new exercise or workout program, don't suddenly ramp up the calories you consume, even if you're trying to gain weight. Your body doesn't like surprises, so keeping things simple in the beginning is the way to go.

Spend the first few days assessing how your body performs during exercise before making changes to your Training Table menu. If you feel energetic all the way through, you don't need additional carbs. If you consistently run out of gas before a workout or practice session is complete, increase your carb intake by adding an extra serving of carbohydrates to two of your daily meals. An easy way? Eat half of a carb-rich banana before your workout and the other half when you complete your routine.

Best Time to Bulk Up

I tell athletes that the best time for them to bulk up is during the off-season. Why? Because off-season workouts are less frequent and less intense. When players aren't burning thousands of calories each week on the practice field, more of the calories they take in can be used to build muscle mass instead of fueling constant physical exertion.

You too may have an "off-season," especially if you live in a northern state and aren't able escape to the Sun Belt for the winter. If for any reason you find yourself laying off sports for weeks or months, take a cue from team athletes and get serious about your weight training during those periods when you have plenty of calories in reserve.

When to Snack. The timing of your day-to-day food intake is also an important consideration when bulking up, especially when doing resistance exercises to build muscle. You'll go at it more efficiently if you eat a mix of carbs and protein 30 minutes before starting. (A fruit smoothie, low-fat chocolate milk, or half a turkey sandwich are examples of good pre-workout snacks.) The food will be digested as you exercise and provide a balance of blood glucose, amino acids, and insulin that combine to rebuild muscle as soon as you finish your regimen.

As you exercise, ask yourself if you have enough energy to get through your activities. If you regularly answer "no," you're probably low on glycogen, which the body synthesizes from glucose. Try eating a banana 15 minutes before you begin, and be sure to drink plenty of fluids before, during, and after exertion.

--- *Take Note* ---

Peel an Apple, Fight Gas

If an apple is your choice for a pre-workout snack (one I wholeheartedly encourage), be sure to peel it before eating. Peeling removes much of the dietary fiber contained in the skin, and here's why you should care: As fiber-rich plant foods are digested they often produce intestinal gas and bloating, which can be a distraction as you exercise or compete. (FYI, the gas is formed when the healthy bacteria in your digestive system try to digest the non-digestible food and create hydrogen, carbon dioxide, and methane.)

So when can a physically active person eat a whole apple, skin and all? Anytime except four hours before you exercise or play sports. Also, remember that if you eat high fiber foods regularly, your body is likely to adapt and produce less gas.

Besides unpeeled apples, fiber-rich foods to avoid for four hours before strenuous exertion include wheat bran; beans, dried peas, and lentils; pears, strawberries, and blueberries; seeds and whole grains and carrots, cucumbers, zucchini, and celery. But don't forget the overall benefit of these foods, which are nutrient-rich and heart healthy. And , flatulence aside, they actually aid digestion.

--- • ---

How Much Should You Weigh?

As discussed in Chapter 1, determining your ideal weight is essential for starting your Training Table program – and, of course, your optimum weight will depend on your age, height, frame size, and physical goals.

Weight estimate alert: The best way to determine your ideal weight is to consult your physician – and, should you play on a college team or professionally, your strength and conditioning coach as well (something you already know). No height-weight chart can equal a personalized evaluation. At the same, you can calculate your own Body Mass Index (as detailed on Chapter 4, "Your Weight Loss/Maintenance Training Table") and also get an idea of healthy weight ranges from other Internet sources and assorted nutrition books.

––– Take Note –––

How the Pros Do It

Professional, collegiate, and other athletes track lean body mass – the mass of the body minus fat. Four methods are typically used, and two of them – underwater weighing and DEXA scans – are quite expensive and are generally available only at universities, diagnostic imaging clinics, hospitals, or research institutions.

Underwater weighing. *Also called hydrostatic weighing, this method measures weight not in pounds but in* percentage of fat to lean muscle. It also takes from 20 to 30 minutes and requires the weighee to be completely submerged for a few minutes.

Bod Pod. While underwater weighing is based on water displacement, this method of measuring lean body mass uses an air displacement device – the Bod Pod, an egg-shaped enclosure in which the weighee undergoes two measurements, each lasting about a minute.

DEXA scans. DEXA, which stands for dual energy X-ray absorptiometry, is used primarily to measure bone density. However, DEXA scans also measure lean body mass, the reason so many athletes undergo the test.

Skinfold calipers. By far the cheapest and most common method of measuring body fat is to use skinfold calipers, which are readily available in athletic stores and online. Calipers measure the subcutaneous fat of several body areas by pinching the skin, and the readings gauge one's percentage of body fat.

___ • ___

For Baby Boomers and Beyond ...

No matter how old you are – a young 54, a still-feel-fine 65 – your exercise options certainly aren't limited to a morning loop around the mega mall. Staying active by regularly exercising or playing sports is vitally important for maintaining your health and quality of life. In fact, lifting weights at this age could actually do you more good than it did when you were at the peak of your physical powers.

You could also swim a few laps at a fitness center or join an aerobics class tailored to people your age. Or get yourself to the court for a game of tennis or join the untold millions of seniors who take to the golf course with even more gusto than they did in their younger years. Whatever you choose to do, just stay active!

If You're the Parent of a Pre-Teen ...

It's never too late to chase the kids off the sofa and show them how to lead healthy lifestyles. Encouraging them to be happily active will help them establish good exercise habits for life. Sign them up for organized sports. Encourage them to play in the yard rather than game on a smartphone or

Wii. Better yet, find things you can do together. Ask them to go for a walk with you after dinner or before school. Go for hikes on the weekend. Go canoeing. Get a family membership at the local family-friendly gym. Just remember that children overheat and dehydrate more quickly than adults do, so have plenty of water at the ready.

--- *Take Note* ---

Pick-Me-Ups for Kids

Does your youngster need a quick pick-me-up? Try a granola bar topped with peanut butter – my daughter's mid-afternoon snack of choice when she was a teen. It's a great source of carbs, fiber, and a little protein and will help hold your child over until the next meal. Another great energy-boosting snack is sliced cantaloupe topped with yogurt and granola.

--- • ---

Chapter 11

Rest to be Your Best

Take It Easy to Play Hard

I f you're like most Americans, you cut corners when it comes to rest. The demands on our time continue to escalate in an ever more hectic world, and we tend to sleep less and less to make room for it all. Unfortunately, the negative effects of sleeplessness reverberate throughout the day and worsen over time.

A good night's sleep is especially important when you stay physically active and play sports, no matter your age. Even missing one full night's sleep can adversely affect your body and mind. Your visual and auditory response times are measurably compromised. You find it difficult to concentrate. You grow irritable more easily. Physically, you tire more quickly, and your athletic performance isn't up to speed because your muscles haven't had a chance to mend properly.

Your Body's Downtime

The busier your body is during the day, the more downtime it needs to repair and rebuild itself. As you drift more deeply into sleep, your body temperature drops, your blood pressure lowers, your pulse stabilizes, and your muscles relax – and the stage is set for your body to "get to work." Blood supplied to your muscles increases, tissue growth and repair take place, and hormones are released into your bloodstream.

Not getting enough sleep can do more damage than you may think, and may pass under an athlete's radar. You may not blame it for the loss of a half step in the 40-yard dash or a lackluster performance in the last set of your tennis match. You might not realize that your deftness with ball, bat, or racquet could improve greatly if you rested more during the day. Truth be told, slim margins such as these often separate the tournament winner from the semi-finalist, the starter from second string, the scholarship athlete from the walk-on.

If your goal is to be the best athlete you can be, you'll want to learn the amount of rest your body requires, then get it.

--- *Take Note* ---

Eddie George At Ease

Day resting was very important to Heisman Trophy winner Eddie George, with whom I worked when he was a two-time Pro-Bowl running back for the Tennessee Titans. Today he heads Eddie George Enterprises (committed to "healthy people, healthy places") and, in 2006, was appointed by Tennessee's governor as the spokesman for GetFitTN.

As I watched George work out and prepare for games, it became clear that he knew how to maximize his athletic talents. He diligently followed the advice of his strength and conditioning coach. He practiced every day with game-day intensity. He made sure his body had the calories, vitamins, and minerals it needed by eating balanced meals and snacks as part of a carefully planned Training Table.

George thought rest just as important as all the preparation. (I often compared his home with a decompression chamber.) After a practice or game, he dimmed the lights, turned off the television and sound system and phone, and put his computer to sleep. This star athlete was more than sold on setting aside time to rest his mind and body – no personal trainer, food coach, or gym membership required!

––– • –––

Counting Sheep (and Hours)

So, just how much sleep do you need to operate at full speed? To find the answer, keep a log of the time you go to bed, the time you wake up, and how you feel when get up. In other words, on days when you bounce out of bed ready to tackle the world, calculate how much sleep you had the night before. Ditto for those mornings when you roll over and hit the snooze button. You'll soon see a correlation between the amount of sleep you get and your energy level and alertness on waking. In turn, you have a better idea of the unique sleep requirements you need each night to awaken fully rested, both mentally and physically. If your log signals that you could use more snooze time, try going to bed at least a half hour earlier each night.

Keep It Quiet, Cool, Dark. Another way to aid sleep is to make your bedroom as slumber-friendly as possible. That means …

- Turning off the phone, television, and anything else that stimulates your brainwaves.
- Making your room as dark as possible, since even a little light can trick your brain into believing it's daytime – and, in turn, to release cortisol, a hormone that promotes alertness.
- Adjust the thermostat so your bedroom stays cool. Your body lowers its temperature as you sleep, so why not help it along?

Sometimes a quiet, pitch-dark room isn't easy to come by, especially in college dormitories and big-city hotels. If this is the case, wear a good-quality sleep mask and use earplugs (experiment with different types of plugs to see which work best for you).

Eat 'n' Drink Smart. If you find it hard to fall asleep at bedtime, ask yourself if you had any caffeine after lunch or used any other stimulants, including nicotine. Both can make getting to sleep difficult, which is, of course, particularly chancy the night before a big game, match, or race. Also, some things you put on your stomach can actually help you get a good night's sleep. Foods high in tryptophan – the amino acid your body uses to create the sleep-inducing substances melatonin and serotonin – are among those to look for. And which foods are good sources of this natural sleep aid? A sampling in alphabetical order includes beans, cheese (especially Swiss and Cheddar), eggs, hazelnuts, hummus, lentils, peanuts, pumpkin seeds, rice, seafood, sesame seeds, soy milk – and, last but not least, turkey. And you thought it was the amount of food gobbled down that makes you sleepy every Thanksgiving!

The Value of Day Resting

I encourage all the athletes I work with to make time to rest before a game. Just as breakfast won't provide you with all the calories and nutrients you need throughout the day, sleeping at night doesn't give your body as much of a break as it needs. And the more athletic you are, the greater your need for rest.

To Nap or Not? "Resting" doesn't necessarily mean sleeping. Even closing your door, turning off the TV and phone, and lying down with your eyes closed for 15 to 20 minutes is helpful. (If you have a pre-game meal, consider having a little lie-down once you've finished eating). For many athletes, such day resting has proved to be extremely beneficial both physically and mentally.

A brief midday nap can help your body prepare for its next workout by relieving stress, which causes your muscles to contract, become tense, and restrict blood flow. Napping or just relaxing and closing your eyes for a short while will not only help your muscles preserve some of their glycogen stores for use later in the day but also can help your body recover from previous exertion.

New Challenges. Still, day napping or day resting may be easier said than done. Technology presents a new wrinkle: Video game-playing, e-mailing, information gathering, and practically every other activity under the sun are standard on smartphones and portable computers, and have a tendency to wind you up. As difficult as it may be, disconnecting yourself long enough to lie still and quiet for a while – or maybe even doze – will do wonders for your energy.

--- *Take Note* ---

Resting During a Workout

There are tremendous benefits in allowing your muscles time to rest and recover – even during a workout, when your heart races to pump oxygen-rich blood to your muscles. By resting for 60 seconds or more between sets, your body has time to replenish the organic compounds required for exercise, such as those found in your body's phosphagen system – one of the three metabolic systems supplying energy for muscle contraction (the other two being the anaerobic glycolysis system and the aerobic system). Phosphagen system compounds are rapidly depleted during exertion, and your minute-long rests between sets allow your body to replenish them and, in the process, make your workouts much more effective.

Another form of rest is also important when exercising: giving the muscles you focused on yesterday the day off from weight training. If you work on different muscle groups each day, you enable your body to maximize its potential as it restores glycogen levels to capacity and makes repairs to muscle tissues.

--- • ---

Chapter 12

Fighting Illness, Healing Injuries

Foods to Help Heal the Hurt

You're looking forward to hitting the lacrosse field on the weekend, but on Tuesday you feel a cold coming on. Or you awaken on the morning of what's planned as a major day of golfing and feel so bloated you wonder if you'll even be able to play. More seriously, months of training for a marathon are all for naught if you come down with a case of the flu, diarrhea, or any other sickness. Whether you're a high school, college, professional, or recreational athlete, you don't want to be sidelined by illness or any other bodily problem.

As pointed out in Chapter 11, Rest to Be Your Best, rest plays a huge role in keeping your body ship-shape. But food is also part of the equation. While no food will cure an illness or heal an injury overnight, certain edibles can provide your body with what it needs to speed the healing process.

Preventing or Treating 20-Plus Sideliners

Following are almost two dozen common health problems that may be putting you off your game. The foods I recommend aren't miracle cures, but rather science-supported strategies for providing the compounds or nutrients your body needs in each instance.

Allergies. (Airborne) See Hay Fever, page 178.

Asthma. While food and drink won't alleviate asthma, some may make you less susceptible to flare-ups. For instance, chicken soup can thin mucus, which tends to block airways – and even the canned version has been shown to help. Many asthma sufferers have found drinking tea to be beneficial. Black, green, or oolong teas contain theophylline, an alkaloid substance used to treat bronchial asthma. In addition, herbal teas made from marshmallow leaf, licorice, horehound, elecampane, or Seneca root have a history of re-lieving bronchial problems. Just don't overdo it; phytochemicals in some herbs interact with pre-scription drugs or cause undesirable side effects when used excessively.

Blisters. Blisters occur when the outer layers of skin separate from the inner layers (usually as a re-sult of friction), and the space between them fills with fluid. While a trainer or coach may help you to treat a blister, it will be up to you to make sure your immune system is ready to help stave off in-fection. For this, I encourage athletes to reach for oranges, guavas, papaya, and cantaloupe – all high in vitamin C, a strong immune-system booster.

Broken Bones. Foods high in calcium, the primary mineral in bones, include tofu, broccoli, almonds, and milk and other dairy products – so eat them up to help fuse a fracture. To help your body ab-sorb calcium, make sure you get plenty of vitamin D, found in eggs, milk, and oily fish. As with any injury rehabilitation, avoid alcohol and tobacco. Both slow the healing process by robbing your body of immune system-friendly vitamin C.

--- *Take Note* ---

Better Bones, Fewer Cramps

Worried about osteoporosis? Plagued by muscle cramps? Turn to lean cuts of beef cooked with little or no fat – say, roasted sirloin. Besides being low in fat (think "heart healthy") lean beef is high in bodybuilding protein and bone-friendly phosphorus. It's also a good source of potassium, which helps stave off muscle cramping during your tennis game or daily jog.

--- • ---

Bruising. Scientists have yet to agree on how effectively nutrition can help to heal a bruise, but many encourage the consumption of leafy dark-green vegetables, broccoli, cauliflower, and liver to boost the body's level of vitamin K. (Bruising occurs when the blood vessels rupture and spill blood beneath the skin, and vitamin K helps blood to clot.) Two other micronutrients – zinc (found in meat and many fortified breakfast cereals) and vitamin C (found in high concentrations in peppers of all sorts, guavas, and citrus fruits) may not only help speed the healing of bruises but may also make your body less prone to bruising.

Burns. To heal burns, including sunburn, your body can't risk a deficiency of the vitamins, minerals, trace elements, and calories it needs to promote healing and tissue repair – in particular, vitamin A, found in dairy products, beef, and liver; vitamin C, whose best sources include peppers, guavas, and citrus fruits; vitamin E, present in eggs, nuts, vegetable oils, leafy dark-green vegetables; and the mineral zinc, found in oysters, red meat, poultry, and fortified breakfast cereals.

If you've suffered a burn and your Training Table is already well balanced, then ramp up the nutrients you take in by adding a daily salad made with a variety of leafy greens, raw vegetables, and legumes (beans peas, lentils, peanuts). Also drink more fluids than usual to help keep your blood plasma from thickening and, in turn, creating additional stress for your body.

Colds and Flu. The first step toward recovering from a cold or the flu is to avoid alcohol, which dilates the blood vessels and makes sinuses and nasal passages feel stuffed up. Step two is to reduce your physical and mental stress – both of which can be relieved by getting plenty of rest. Third, reach for foods rich in zinc, a mineral that can shorten a cold's duration. Good zinc sources include wheat germ, dried peas and beans, oysters, seafood, meat, poultry, dairy products, and tofu.

Constipation. You aren't going to be able to play or run your best if you have difficulty emptying your bowels. When athletes are constipated, I encourage them to increase their fluid intake and to eat foods rich in insoluble fiber as quickly as possible – foods like figs, prunes, brown rice, raisins, and whole-wheat products. In addition, foods high in magnesium, such as spinach, chocolate, and avocados, can act as a gentle laxative.

Cramps (Muscular). These painful spasms are often the result of overexertion and fatigue. Though typically short-lived, they interfere with any athletic activity. Massage and stretching the afflicted area will help the muscle to relax. Cramps are often a metabolic response to a depletion of electrolytes (see "Electrolytes Keep You Charged" in Chapter 9, Hydration, Hydration, Hydration.) Typically, electrolytes are in ample supply in your body but become scarce after 90 minutes or more of vigorous exertion, or in less time if you sweat heavily. At the beginning of extended periods of activity, drink 5 to 10 ounces of water every 10 to 20 minutes. Then, as you approach the end of the first hour of exertion, start drinking an electrolyte-supplemented sports drink. To further lessen the chances of muscle cramping and speed relief, do the following:

- Increase your potassium intake by eating foods rich in this mineral – bananas, dried apricots, walnuts, and sunflower seeds.
- If you sweat a lot (therefore lowering your sodium level and making you more susceptible to cramping) eat salty foods such as pretzels, pickles, and deli meats prior to exercise or play.
- Avoid nicotine and caffeine, both of which restrict blood flow.

Cramps (Menstrual). Some studies suggest that calcium can help relieve symptoms associated with a woman's menstrual cycle, including abdominal cramping. Low levels of calcium, whose absorption is regulated by the hormone estrogen, seem to coincide with elevated levels of discomfort for women. Accordingly, drink an extra glass of calcium-enriched milk each day. Also take in more vitamin D (present in egg yolks, milk, cheese, and other dairy products) to facilitate the absorption of calcium. And don't forget sunlight. Soaking up as little as 10 minutes each day (depending on its intensity in your region) will make your skin produce vitamin D in response to ultraviolet radiation.

Dehydration. See Chapter 9, Hydration, Hydration, Hydration.

Depression. If you have a mild case of the blues, seek out foods containing tryptophan, an amino acid that promotes a healthy nervous system. Tryptophan is common in such foods as roasted turkey breast, yellow fin tuna, soybeans, and shrimp. Also helpful is the micronutrient choline, often classed as a B vitamin, which promotes healthy brain function; good choline sources include oatmeal and members of the cabbage family – broccoli, cauliflower, Brussels sprouts, kale, collards, and white or red cabbage. Avoid both caffeine, which can cause mood swings as well as insomnia, and alcohol, which is a depressant.

Diarrhea. Obviously, digestive irregularities including diarrhea hamper an athlete's performance. Although this troublesome ailment won't be remedied by a particular food, it's imperative to drink water to replace large amounts of fluids lost to diarrhea. Also be sure to avoid spicy foods, caffeine (a diuretic), milk, and high-sugar drinks, all of which can aggravate the condition.

Ear Infections. Besides being uncomfortable, ear infections can create balance problems. If you feel an infection coming on, eat lots of fruits and vegetables – particularly citrus fruits and peppers and other plant foods rich in vitamin C – to give a boost to your immune system. Things to avoid include saturated fats and foods high in salts, which can lead to an excess of inner-ear fluid and increase the level of discomfort.

Gas. Like other digestive conditions, excessive gas can cause discomfort and distract you from your game. To help prevent it, limit your intake of foods your body has difficulty digesting. For most people, this means beans and all members of the cabbage family. You may find that eating acidophilis-culture yogurt each day will help your body to process hard-to-digest food more effectively. Fennel seeds and caraway seeds can help ease flatulence, whether they're sprinkled on food or taken in tea. Avoid carbonated drinks and chewing gum, both of which cause you to swallow air. Athletes with even slight lactose intolerance should avoid milk, lest they start feeling a little gassy.

Hay Fever. Eating foods high in omega-3 fatty acids can often minimize the effects of this seasonal allergy, thanks to omega-3's ability to reduce inflammation in the respiratory system. Cold-water fish including salmon, mackerel, albacore tuna, and sardines are all rich in omega-3, as are tofu and other soy products.

Hives. This skin rash is usually caused by an unusual sensitivity to a normally harmless substance, whether it is breathed in, eaten, or comes into contact with your skin. The allergic reaction causes the release of histamines, which can produce the itchy skin blotches typical of hives. Hives can also be caused by stress. Eating foods high in niacin, including whole-grain products, fish, and poultry, often reduce the body's release of histamines, curtailing the itching and swelling associated with hives. If stress is the cause, add food with high levels of tryptophan (among them turkey and soy products) to your menu.

Indigestion. Used medicinally for thousands of years, ginger helps quell indigestion and nausea. This Asian root also comes in multiple forms, including fresh gingerroot shavings, ginger ale, ginger beer, ginger tea, ginger snap cookies, and crystallized (candied) ginger. Avoidance is the best remedy for preventing indigestion and heartburn during athletic activity. Among the foods and beverages to shun are greasy burgers and fries; spicy foods; citrus juices; coffee (with the exception of decaf); and beer, wine, and spirits. Tobacco, too, can contribute to a case of indigestion.

Inflammation. The swelling and pain of muscle and joint inflammation are all too familiar to avid athletes. Foods rich in omega-3 fatty acids, especially cold-water fish such as salmon, sardines, mackerel, albacore tuna, and halibut help reduce the symptoms, as do tofu and other soy products. Eating a handful of crystallized ginger every two days can also bring relief, thanks to its large quantities of a natural anti-inflammatory compound called shogoals.

––– *Take Note* –––

Gary's Chronic Knee Pain

It looked as if Gary, an NFL player 12 years out from his glory days, would have to resort to surgery to ease the chronic pain he felt in both knees. His physician provided moderate relief through prescription anti-inflammatories, yet it was a less invasive and no-cost measure that did the trick.

That measure was weight loss. Gary still weighed what he did in his pro days – and too much poundage means extra stress to the knees. Through low-impact exercise and an exacting Training Table, Gary lost 40 pounds in 10 months. He also felt such relief that his physician saw no need for him to undergo knee surgery.

––– • –––

Mononucleosis. Mononucleosis, an acute viral infection that typically lasts for four to six weeks, can sideline any athlete because fatigue can linger even after the other symptoms (fever, sore throat, and swollen lymph glands) have subsided. To help your body fight fatigue, drink plenty of water and other fluids and eat lots of fruits and vegetables to help boost both energy and the immune system.

Osteoporosis. Women and men alike begin to lose bone mass around the age of 30. This bone thinning, called osteoporosis, makes bones more susceptible to fractures. To strengthen bones, eat foods high in calcium (dairy and soy products, dark green leafy vegetables, legumes) and vitamin D (milk, fatty fish), and eat them regularly. Calcium is the raw material your body uses to repair and rebuild bones, and vitamin D helps the body to absorb it. A non-dietary way to lessen the decline in bone density is to regularly perform resistance exercises (see "Aerobic vs. Resistance Exercise" in Chapter 10, "Working Out, Weighing In.")

Sore Throat. A sore throat is typically caused by a viral or bacterial infection, sinus drainage, pollen, or smoke. Regardless of the source of the irritation, foods rich in vitamin C (citrus juices, guavas, peppers, parsley, broccoli) and zinc (oysters, red meat, poultry, and fortified breakfast cereals) can help hasten relief. If swallowing solid food is particularly uncomfortable, try a vitamin-packed fruit smoothie, which will not only be easier to swallow but also will help boost your immune system.

--- *Take Note* ---

Guava: The Oft-Overlooked Superstar

Guava, a tropical fruit native to Latin America, is low on the average consumption-per-year ladder but sky-high in a number of important nutrients. Here's a comparison of guava and the orange, drawn from the USDA National Nutrition Database. A hundred grams of raw common guava (the most widely available) supplies ...

- *Almost four times more vitamin C than the equivalent amount of navel orange*
- *Two-and-a-half times the potassium*
- *Twice as much magnesium*

In addition, the guava's content of the healthful phytochemical known as lycopene (a caretenoid) is off the charts: 5,204 international units (IU) compared to zero for all types of oranges.

--- • ---

Urinary Tract Infections. Long used to prevent urinary tract infections, cranberry juice has what it takes. The high volume of hippuric acid and fructose in cranberries helps to keep E. coli bacteria from adhering to bladder and urethra tissues. Undiluted, unsweetened cranberry juice is considerably more preventive than the sweetened variety. Increasing your daily water intake will also help to prevent urinary tract infections.

Vaginal Yeast Infections. Vaginal yeast infections – also called vaginitis – are typically caused by an imbalance of "good" bacteria and microorganisms inside a woman's body. Some women experience symptomatic relief by eating acidophilus-culture yogurt daily and cutting down on sugary foods, which can promote the growth of yeast.

Eating to Win with America's #1 Food Coach
is available for all e-readers, including the iPad,
the Kindle, and the Nook.